HERBS &
INFLUENZA

*How herbs used in the
1918 Flu Pandemic can be
effective in ANY Pandemic*

KATHY ABASCAL JD, RH (AHG)

Tigana Press
Vashon, WA 98070

Photographs:
Gelsemium sempervirens (cover image) Ralph Lyon, 228-234-1137
Asclepias tuberosa (back cover image) Holly Shull Vogel
Trolley: Courtesy of the National Archives & Records Admin.
Nurses: Courtesy of Library of Congress
Flu Ward: Courtesy of the National Museum of Health & Meicine
Eclectics: Courtesy of Henrietta Kress
Illustrations: Kathy Abascal

Herbs & Influenza: How herbs used in the 1918 Flu Pandemic
can be effective in ANY pandemic
Second revised edition

ISBN number: 0-9788586-8-9

The author and Tigana Press disclaim any liability in connection with the use of information contained in this book. For
additional information please contact
Tigana Press, P.O. Box 1528, Vashon WA 98070
email tiganapress@gmail.com or visit www.TQIDiet.com

DEDICATION

To Holly Shull Vogel who keeps me and my work flowing and organized.

To Daniel Klein for motivating me to update this book.

To David Hinchman of Vashon Print & Design without whose skill & knowledge & help this book would not have made it to print.

Preface to the second edition of Herbs & Influenza.

When this book was written back in 2005-2006, H1N1 (aka bird flu) was looming as a potential pandemic flu virus. The world found itself unprepared for the disruption and misery a pandemic with the ability to spread quickly while causing many people serious complications and death. The book details the steps taken at the time to cope with that pandemic (such as stockpiling antiviral medications), none of which looked especially promising at the time.

In the approximately fifteen years that have passed since the book came out, pandemic preparedness has actually decreased. Today, as a new virus rears its head as a pandemic threat, we are discovering that we today are actually more vulnerable to pandemic viruses. We continue to need to know how to use both our diet and herbs to help us cope with potential pandemic viruses. This need is what has motivated me to print an updated version of Herbs & Influenza.

The majority of the book – how herbs were used in the Pandemic of 1918 - has of course not changed at all. So, to expedite this new printing, I decided to present specific information on what has changed since the book's original publication in an introductory update.

Kathy Abascal
Vashon, Washington
March 2020

UPDATES

Introduction
(page 9)

In 2006, experts agreed the world was ill prepared for a pandemic. People traveled widely guaranteeing that a virus could spread quickly across the world. Health care was streamlined and lacked necessary medical equipment to handle significant increases in demand.

In 2020, our economy is more global than ever. For instance, in 2006, about 850 million tourists traveled the world. In 2018, 1.32 billion did. The world's population has grown and we have more under- and poorly-nourished people as well as far more people coping with chronic ailments that predispose them to viral complications. Our healthcare has continued to be streamlined and more efficient "bed management" and a higher "bed turnover rate" is a health care goal used to increase profits. Just as in 2006, the existing hospital respirators are in use and hospital beds will be in short supply if there is any uptick in need. In Wuhan, the center of the recent outbreak, two Coronovirus hospitals were built in just over a week. They add-ed another 16 hospitals just to cope with their outbreak. The US has neither funds nor plans to accomplish anything similar. In 2020 in the US, just as in 2006, very few are going receive the intensive hospital care that may be needed to treat the com-plications of a pandemic virus. The original Introduction on page9 remains as pertinent today as it did when it was written and I hope you take the time to read it.

WHAT IS INFLUENZA?
(page 11)

Bird flu did not become a 1918 flu type pandemic. It does, however, continue to simmer amongst the masses of caged and immune suppressed fowl worldwide, and continues to be closely watched because it could at any moment mutate into a troubling virus. As a result, the details on how bird flu might manifest remains quite relevant. After describing the flu virus, the book details how MDs successfully used herbs to treat victims of the 1918 pandemic. Their treatments were symptom rather than disease based. They did not have a standard treatment for influenza but instead administered herbs chosen specifically for a type of cough or a type of fever or constellation of symptoms.

At the moment, we are coping with a novel Corona virus, SARS-CoV-2, instead of a flu virus. There are hundreds of Corona viruses (CoVs) that can cause fever, respiratory problems, and sometimes GI issues. The common cold is a corona virus and many corona strains are annoying but not dangerous. However, some like MERS (Middle Eastern respiratory syndrome) and SARS (severe acute respiratory syndrome) attach in the lungs and bronchial tubes causing more serious infections often with high fatality rates. The strain of concern in 2020 is named SARS-CoV-2 because it genetically close to SARS.

CoVid-19 is the disease someone infected with SARS-CoV-2 gets. It often causes a fever and dry cough with the ability to progress rather quickly to shortness of breath, pneumonia, organ and respiratory failure if untreated.[1] Reports from Wuhan, the epicenter of this infection said the early CoVid-19 cases experienced a dry cough and fever for about 6 days with increasing shortness of breath that typically required hospital-

1 I will for convenience and brevity sometimes call both the SARS-CoV-2 virus and Covid-19 illness as Covid-19.

ization on day 7 and intensive care respiratory support including mechanical ventilation by day 8.

Because Eclectic doctors in 1918 selected herbs for specific symptom patterns and particular problems, their herbs should work for any virus that triggers those symptoms. In other words, treatments used for the 1918 influenza will work as well for a strain of bird flu or a strain of corona virus if they cause the same symptoms. That's why the Eclectic treatments are relevant in any pandemic. At the end of this update I will discuss the remedies that I think might be most useful in coping with CoVid-19 if it continues to spread and conventional medical help is not available.

CONVENTIONAL TREATMENTS FOR PANDEMIC INFLUENZA
(Page 21)

Vaccines

There currently are no vaccines for MERS or SARS or the corona virus causing the CoVid-19 illness. However, much work is underway to create one for this strain. This has its downsides. Vaccine manufacturers have obtained near complete freedom from liability for pandemic vaccines under virtually all circumstances. The desire to create a new vaccine before the epidemic is too far gone (or blows over) creates pressure, not only to save lives that might be lost in a full-blown pandemic but also out of the prospect of huge economic gain. The specter of enormous profits for a timely new vaccine, combined with the complexity of viruses, and the freedom from accountability, increases the likelihood of both mistakes and of cutting of corners when testing the effectiveness and potential side effects of a novel vaccine. The discussion of vaccines beginning on page 21 contains additional issues that compound those problems and make a new vaccine that may become mandatory as scary as the pandem ic virus itself.

Antiviral drugs

The US ultimately spent over 1.3 billion stockpiling antiviral drugs when bird flu appeared. Worldwide stockpiling and private hoarding ran into yet more billions of dollars. The drugs purchased for the potential bird flu outbreak were set to expire after 5 years. When 5 years passed without a pandemic, governments did not dump the stockpiles but instead simply extended the "use by" date another 5 years.[2]

In 2014, the Cochrane Collaboration concluded that the antiviral drugs were a complete waste of money. At best, the drugs shortened flu symptoms by about half a day (from 7 to 6.3 days) but did not cut hospital admissions or lessen complications of the drug.[3] The drugs instead caused nausea and vomiting in 4-5% of those taking them. As well, there are reports of neuropsychiatric side effects (e.g., abnormal behavior, altered mental status, hallucinations, delirium and suicide) in young people. Japan, whose population as of 2019 had taken more than 3/4ths of all Tamiflu, found those reported complications sufficiently concerning that it banned the use of Tamiflu by teenagers.

Despite serious questions about the effectiveness of

2 A military study recently found that most drugs actually remain fully potent for at least a decade past their use by date so this likely was harmless but does suggest we should revisit the advice we consumers get to discard drugs as soon as they are past their "use by" date.
3 The Cochrane review analyzed 20 studies on Tamiflu and 26 on Relenza and found they did not prevent complications in people with "regular" flu. There is no data on how these antivirals could possibly be effective in a flu strain with a far stronger ability to cause complications.

these antiviral drugs, governments globally continue to stock pile them. Although they question the validity of the many studies showing a lack of effectiveness, antivirals continue to be stockpiled primarily out of fear of public unrest if the country is faced with a pandemic lacking any treatment options.

Currently, a number of new antiviral drugs are coming that no doubt will be added to our stockpiles. Baloxavir, licensed in the US and Japan in 2018, belongs to a new type of antivirals, the polymerase inhibitors. So far it seems no better at reducing flu symptoms or complications than either Tamiflu or Relenza. However, it may be better at somewhat limiting viral shedding which affects spreading of the virus. Pimodivir and Favipiravir, two other polymerase inhibitors, are also moving toward market. Pimodivir is in a phase III trial and, if licensed for seasonal influenza, would definitely be considered for pandemic use. Favipiravir is already part of the Japanese stockpile but, because it may cause birth defects, it will be used only if resistance to other antivirals develops.

These antivirals, however, are neither created nor licensed for use against a SARS type virus, such as the one responsible for CoVid-19.

OUR PLAN FOR THE PANDEMIC
(page 29)

The book details the Pandemic Plan put in place back in 2006. In the interim, no progress has been made to improve our actual ability to handle a pandemic and, in fact, in recent years we have actually moved in the opposite direction since president Trump took office:

The 2021 budget, introduced 11 days after the World Health Organization declared Covid-19 to be a public health emergency, reduced the Center for Disease Control spending 16% from 2020. Although they have been countered by Congress each time, each of Trump's budgets have called for cuts to CDC spending.

The president fired the person responsible for coordinating administration efforts to combat infectious disease at the Na-tional Security Council. As one writer explained: The president fired the pandemic specialist in this country two years ago in 2018.

The Trump administration has consistently called for deep cuts to USAID's (United States Agency for International Development) budget. This agency runs the Emerging Pandemic Threats program to help detect and control infectious diseases that emerge in animals and people before they become significant threats to human health.

For the last three years, the Trump administration has sought to cut funding for NIH (National Institutes of Health). This agency has the primary responsibility for biomedical and public health research.

For the fourth straight year, sizeable reductions in federal research spending is proposed. In the first two years of the Trump administration, 1600 scientists left their government positions.

Even as Covid-19 spreads globally, the president takes the position that the coronavirus will miracu-lously disappear by April and is relying on 'warm weather' to end the spread of the virus.

WHAT LIES IN STORE FOR COVID-19?

There are a number of possible outcomes for this new virus:

1. CoVid-19 may continue to spread rapidly, overwhelming health care resources, disrupting commerce, and causing much illness and many deaths in the near future.
2. CoVid-19 may be contained by current efforts to limit travel and increase hand washing hygiene. Plus, the move toward warmer weather and improved levels of vitamin D in the Northern Hemisphere may increase the public's immunity to the disease.
3. CoVid-19 might mutate into a less threatening virus and simply become another strain of a common cold.
4. CoVid-19 might seem to disappear as spring arrives but then, come fall, roar back in the same or a more virulent form, just as the 1918 flu did. This scenario would then have many coping simultaneously with a difficult pandemic Corona virus and an annual flu strain.

MY THOUGHTS ON PREPARING FOR COVID-19

The initial symptoms of CoVid-19 are usually a fever and dry cough that soon begins to create a shortness of breath. In complicated cases, this quickly develops into a level of shortness of breath requiring hospitalization and very quickly intensive care and respiratory support that may require mechanical ventilation. The statistics on CoVid-19 are currently all over the place but it was reported that 90% of the early cases in Wuhan hospitals could not breathe spontaneously and that 45-65% of those treated in ICU worsened and died.

One research study posited that the virus is finding a way to move through the blood brain barrier and disrupt the respiratory centers of the brain, leading to death.[4] It suggested that some type antiviral therapy should be carried out as early as possible to block the virus from accessing respiratory centers in the brain using inhalation of antiviral agents as the first treatment choice at the early stage of infection. Steroids were contraindicated as they appeared to accelerate the replication of the virus in neurons.

As I consider this, my thought is to use some herbs to reign in the virus in those initial days of fever and cough while trying to move antiviral compounds into the lung tissue by inhalation.

The remedies that I think might be most useful in the early stages are:

1. *Eupatorium Perfoliatum* L.
(Page 61)

This herb has a long use in many cultures for colds, sore throats, pneumonia, and pleurisy. It is diaphoretic, meaning it will help bring down a fever. It was used by many as a preventative by some in 1918. Boneset is probably my favorite herb to use when I've been around people I suspect are shedding the flu virus.

Unfortunately, pyrrolizidine alkaloids (PAs) were identified in boneset. While some PAs are very liver toxic, those found in boneset do not appear to be. Nonetheless, out of fear and an excess of caution, it is virtually impossible to find boneset tincture on the market. It is, however, a plant that is easy to grow so if CoVid-19 takes a break over the summer, or if you want to prepare for next year's flu season, you might want to

---

4 One young medical graduate student who survived in Wuan said she had to stay awake and consciously breathe during intensive care. She said that "if she fell asleep, she might die because she had lost her natural breath."

grow it and make your own medicine. I imagine that many private practitioners who incorporate botanical medicine in their practice may still dispense boneset for appropriate use.

2. *Asclepia Tuberosa* L.
(Page 69)
This beautiful plant has a long and varied use for dry and constricted coughs. It is thought to improve lung function, and has been used to reduce fevers. It was considered an excellent remedy for colds – strains of Corona viruses. The Eclectics often combined it with other herbs and I would probably combine it with lobelia.

3. *Lobelia* spp.
(Page 100)
This herb was used in small doses for colds with a dry irritative cough. A few drops of it could be combined with Asclepias for that cough. I have used small doses of lobelia on the few occasions where I have had the flu and it very effectively reduced the painful constriction of my chest.

4. *Echinacea* spp.
(Page 111)
Echinacea is a pleasant herb that has been shown to help quiet the excessive inflammatory cytokine production many viruses cause. It was a prominent remedy in fevers. One Eclectic physician recommended simply giving Echinacea as part of treatment from beginning to end when it came to coughs.

5. Chest Applications
(Page 153)
CoVid-19 has a tendency to move quickly deep into the respiratory tract and relatively quickly disrupt breathing.

Studies out of Wuhan show rapid build-up of excess fluid in the lungs that occurred even in asymptomatic patients. Delivering medications (be they herb or pharmaceutical) becomes difficult as the fluid in the lungs impedes the movement of those heal-ing compounds from the blood stream into the lung tissues. As well, the study mentioned above suggested that the use of inhalant antiviral compounds might prevent the virus from moving into the brain, deemed to be the possible cause of the most serious complications.

Chest applications and inhalants deliver antiviral vol-atiles that have been shown to be able to move through and into fluid filled lungs. I recommend spending time reading the section on Eclectic chest applications. My first choice will be a variety of Vicks Vaporub or similar products that contain eucalyptus, menthol, and camphor. Vicks comes as a chest rub, for use in a vaporizer, and in tablet form for use in the shower. I recommend starting these applications at the first sign of a potential viral symptom, remembering to cover both front and back of the chest. I also plan on making the powder of Lobe-lia but the onion poultice or juniper pomade described in this chapter also make good sense. Because these applications are going to be messy, you might want to stock up on inexpensive t-shirts and cotton gauze.

6. Quieting the Immune System.

When I wrote the first edition of this book, I was a practicing professional herbalist. I remain an herbalist but no longer practice. Over time, I realized that, while herbs are fab-ulous tools, they did not prevent and often did not cure illness. In a desire to learn more about health, my research and prac-tice moved steadily from herbs toward diet and food. I focused on inflammation and over time developed a diet that quiets chronic inflammation, the TQI Diet.

In any pandemic, even the worst of the worst, many do

not get sick. Some even work closely with sick people but do not get sick. Our goal should be to be one of those who do not succumb to the pandemic virus. If we cannot achieve that, we should work on being one of those who develops a mild case using the herbs and chest applications as needed.
How to do that? Start quieting the excess chronic inflammation you carry right now by eating well.

We assume that the elderly are frail and that their frailty is why they often end up hospitalized with pneumonia after a bout of the flu or even die from a "regular" strain of flu. One study, however, challenged this view. It looked at a group of elderly who ate and lived well and found that their levels of inflammatory cytokines were no higher than those of young healthy people. When they got the flu, they did not suffer any more complications than the young did. Why?

When we are exposed to a novel or difficult virus, our immune system sets off a cascade of inflammatory cytokines that actually cause most of the negative symptoms that we associate with that virus. In pandemic flu, the resulting cytokine storm is what kills, not the flu virus itself. It is our immune system's overreaction to the flu. In an average cold, it is not the corona virus that cause your nose to run and you to cough, it is your immune response to the virus that does. What we know is this: If you are not inflamed, your immune system's reaction will not result in such intense symptoms. At most you will suffer a milder case of what is going around. If on the other hand, you start off inflamed, your cytokine levels are high on a regular basis. Then you get exposed to a novel virus. The additive effect of your preexisting inflammation with the new inflammation will send you over the edge, into pneumonia and possible organ dysfunction and death.

The very best thing you can do to avoid CoVid-19 is not to wash your hands or quit picking your nose (though both are important things to work on doing). The best thing you could do: Eat to quiet inflammation which means stop indulging in foods and beverages that stress your immune system. Instead eat a lot of nutrient rich foods so your body has the tools to function well. And there is no doubt in my mind that the best way to this is to visit my website, TQIDiet.com, and either take a class or buy the TQI Diet books, read the blogs, and begin to care for your body as the precious thing it really is.

TABLE OF CONTENTS

PREFACE

Influenza is coming this fall, as it does every fall. This year, however, we are being warned that the coming flu may be the "Bird Flu" or another pandemic strain of influenza. This flu will be extraordinarily contagious and much more deadly than the usual seasonal flu virus.

Herbal medicine has a long history of easing flu symptoms and preventing potentially fatal complications. Herbs have been relied on to ease the aches and pains of the "ordinary" seasonal flu. They also worked well in the world-wide flu pandemic of 1918 as well as the lesser known pandemic of 1889 in which 40% of the United States total population came down with the flu. I have explored in depth the history of herbal influenza treatments, and I am convinced that herbs are an important resource for any type of influenza, seasonal or pandemic.

The information on herbal influenza treatments is of great importance because, unfortunately, conventional medicine has a limited ability to treat influenza. While governmental officials convey the impression that sufficient preparations are diligently proceeding, our preparation is inadequate. I hope I am wrong about how tragically inadequate our plans are, in both substance and scope, but experts agree that presently we are not ready to cope with pandemic influenza. I believe that to be truly ready, we must use all available resources. Our planning must include taking into account how herbal medicines can make our preparation more effective.

The first edition of this book contains all of the substantive material I could locate on herbal treatments for pandemic influenza. I am satisfied with its accuracy but the book has less in the way of illustrations and other design elements than I would have liked. However, I decided to proceed to print quickly just in case this coming season is when the next pandemic flu hits.

Kathy Shull Abascal
Vashon, Washington
August 2006

INTRODUCTION

In 1918, influenza circled the globe several times, infecting vast numbers and killing millions of people, including young, healthy adults. The descriptions of its victims are vivid and linger in the mind: Six thousand soldiers were crammed into a hospital set up for twelve hundred. They lay sick and dying in halls and on porches without nursing care because many nurses were sick and dying as well. Bodies filled the morgue and spilled out into surrounding areas. And the disease was not gentle, even mild cases brought much pain, weakness, and lingering coughs.

Many experts say we are overdue for another influenza pandemic, and all agree that the world is ill prepared for it. People travel widely today, and a highly infectious influenza strain would spread quickly to every corner of the world. Our hospital systems are streamlined, and there is not enough equipment or medicine to treat an outbreak that is predicted to rapidly infect 40% of the population. Virtually all existing hospital respirators are already in use, and hospital beds will be in extremely short supply. In fact, preparedness plans have already identified the groups that will be given first access to treatment. Other groups, such as the elderly, will be at the end of a very long line. Most people will not receive any treatment, let alone cutting edge treatments, should any effective new treatments develop. So it makes sense to consider whether plant medicines can be used either as a part of a primary treatment plan or a fall-back position in the next influenza pandemic when conventional treatments may be unavailable.

It is not far fetched to seriously consider the usefulness of plants in a pandemic. Contrary to common belief, herbs were used effectively in the 1918 pandemic. A group of American physicians, the Eclectics, used medicinal plants to treat their influenza patients. They consistently reported that their remedies successfully eased symptoms and averted fatal complications in most of their patients. Only 0.6% of patients treated with herbs died in an epidemic that otherwise killed at least 2.8% of those who got sick with the flu. Until now, their remedies have remained buried and unread in old, obscure alternative medical journals and textbooks. These treatments have not been looked at seriously due, in large part, to the politics of medicine. With the threat of a pandemic looming, it is time to set aside preconceptions about the usefulness of plants and examine these remedies because they may be all we have in the next pandemic.

This book is intended both for lay people and professionals. It describes pandemic flu strains, and the current treatment options available. The plants the Eclectics used, as well as how they chose and dosed their remedies, are then described in detail. Some of the plants are very common and could be used as a home treatment. Others are less common, and require a trained professional to determine the correct time of administration and dose. Understanding the Eclectic treatment of influenza will enable anyone to have some remedies at hand to ease influenza symptoms. It will allow practitioners to become familiar with how to best use plant remedies in a fierce pandemic. Finally, the reports and insights of the Eclectic physicians are a resource for contemporary scientists interested in investigating influenza treatments.

What Is Influenza?

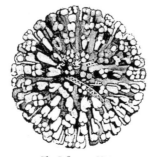

The Influenza Virus

Flu Viruses

Influenza viruses are tiny, minimalist beings that use other creatures to replicate their structures. Influenza viruses have a core of genetic material surrounded by a protective protein layer, and an envelope studded with protein-sugar spikes. These spikes help the virus invade cells but they also trigger immune responses in the host. Some of the spikes are hemaglutinin in different forms, H1 to H16. Some of the spikes are neuramidase, N1 to N9. Different influenza viral strains are identified based on the types of spikes on their envelope. Thus, the avian flu is called "H5N1" based on its studs. The 1918 flu virus was an "H1N1" strain.

Viruses are highly mutable creatures. They change their envelope studs constantly, creating new shapes that immune systems do not recognize or cannot effectively control. Flu vaccines change each year in an attempt to "match" the currently circulating strain.

Virtually every mammal has its own strains of influenza. Sometimes a strain will mutate into a highly lethal form, as the avian flu has, causing a high death rate in its target species, in this case birds. Occasionally, mutations enable the virus to infect a new species, and those changes cause a high death rate in the new, "naïve" species. These mutations may occur more easily when a virus infects a new host already suffering from its own strain of flu. That is, a pig already sick with pig flu also gets a bird flu. These two viruses then commingle forming a new strain that is more lethal to pigs and perhaps also able to move to, and between, humans or other species. Species jumping is not a one-way street. In 1998, a human virus moved into the pig population causing widespread disease.[1]

Human flu pandemics have probably occurred since man domesticated animals. Species jumping occurs more easily when different species live closely together. Thus, the bird flu victims usually come from households that raised chickens and fighting cocks in their yards, where children were exposed to chicken waste in the dirt and probably water, and where people handled diseased animals and may have eaten uncooked foods.

So far, the avian strain has only rarely moved from person to person. Some experts believe that avian viruses change into a type that can move from human to human after first infecting pigs, and many of our influenza viruses have originated in China where pigs, birds, and humans live in close quarters. But species jumping can occur anywhere, at any time. In many countries, the trend is to separate livestock from people but in the United States, factory farming crowds animals into small areas in relatively close proximity both to other animals and densely populated areas. This can provide a hospitable environment for commingling between strains.

THERE IS FLU, AND THERE IS DEADLY FLU

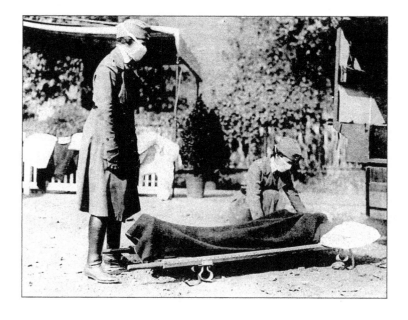

Every year, new flu strains cross the globe. These strains cause the well known discomforts of fever, muscle aches, headaches, and tightness in the chest. They make many people miserable for a few days but usually pass quickly. The flu is often more dangerous for the elderly, the very young, and those with weak immune systems (such as people with HIV or AIDS, transplant recipients or those undergoing cancer treatment). These groups may suffer deadly secondary infections, such as pneumonia, after a bout of the flu. Flu strains that create pandemics are different because they are more infectious and cause more deaths.

Many influenza pandemics have a high morbidity, that is, a high percentage of the population comes down with the flu. In the 1889-1890 pandemic, 40% of the population came down with the flu. Many pandemics, however, did not cause a high mortality, that is, a high death rate. The 1918 flu was unique because it had a high morbidity *and* a high mortality rate. The avian flu, so far, has a low morbidity because it is not transmitted well from person to person, but has a very high mortality rate, right now at about 60%.

Pandemic Influenza Symptoms

Influenza expresses itself in many different ways. Each pandemic had unique symptoms that troubled patients and physicians. In the pandemic of 1889-1890, the flu expressed itself in distinct and varied ways.

(1) Influenza with respiratory symptoms was most common. It began with a chill or a severe head cold with sneezing and weakness. A persistent cough followed that was usually paroxysmal and violent. Patients spit up copious amounts of lumps of greenish-yellow sputum, and their coughing fits left them exhausted. Bronchitis and broncho-pneumonia patches were common but some suffered pneumonia or pleurisy. The illness lasted less than two weeks in uncomplicated cases but left the patients weak and frail for much longer, in some cases for months. The greatest danger in this type of influenza was the potential for severe pulmonary complications that could be fatal.

(2) Influenza with nerve symptoms did not cause cold symptoms, and often only produced a slight fever. However,

its "atrocious feature" was the intense almost unbearable pain in the head, back, joints, and limbs. Depression was characteristic. Some patients went into delirium and some committed suicide to escape the intense pain. Severe cases suffered pathological changes to the brain, abscesses and paralysis could occur, and many patients were left with more or less permanent depression and dementia.

(3) Influenza with gastrointestinal symptoms was marked by copious watery diarrhea with nausea, vomiting, and severe abdominal pain. The diarrhea was resistant to most diarrhea remedies, and could persist for three to four weeks.

(4) Influenza with febrile symptoms was rare. Patients with this type of influenza suffered a fever that lasted for several weeks. The fever sometimes waxed and waned with intermittent chills.

(5) Finally, influenza with inflammatory symptoms was dominated by severe rheumatoid pains in the joints. Unlike rheumatoid arthritis, however, it did not cause permanent damage to the joints.[2]

The 1918 influenza was different from the 1889 pandemic strain because patient symptoms did not fall into the discrete categories of influenza described above. Instead, patients suffered from many different and difficult types of symptoms.

John Barry's book "The Great Influenza" contains some vivid descriptions of the 1918 pandemic. In complicated and usually fatal cases, the symptoms were striking and frightening. Their flu caused extreme muscular pain, severe headaches, and rapidly attacked the lungs. Many turned a dark, dusky indigo blue as their lungs failed to receive oxygen, coagulation defects shut down major organs and caused blood to spurt from noses, ears, mouths, and other orifices. The 1918 flu could cause death quickly. One South African doctor reported getting on a street car only to have the conductor fall over dead. In the next three miles, six passengers and the street car driver died; the doctor ended up walking home. [3]

Mostly, people in 1918 suffered extremely unpleasant symptoms for several days and then recovered in about ten days. "[B]ut in a minority of cases, and not just in a tiny minority, the virus manifested itself in an influenza that did not follow normal patterns, that was unlike any influenza ever reported...Generally in the Western world, the virus demonstrated extreme virulence or led to pneumonia in from 10 to 20 percent of all cases. ... To those who suffered a violent attack, there often was pain, terrific pain, and the pain could come from almost anywhere.... Extreme earaches were common. One physician observed that otitis media – inflammation of the middle ear marked by pain, fever, and dizziness –'developed with surprising rapidity, and rupture of the drum membrane was observed at times in a few hours after the onset of pain.'...In U.S. army cantonments, from 5 percent to 15 percent of all men hospitalized suffered from epistaxis – bleeding from the nose – as with hemorrhagic viruses such as Ebola. There were many reports that blood sometimes spurted from the nose with enough power to travel several feet." [4]

Barry describes an influenza outbreak aboard a naval vessel: "The sailors were covered with blood mostly from nosebleeds although a few had coughed the blood up, others had bled from their ears. Some coughed so hard that autopsies later would show they had torn apart abdominal muscles and rib cartilage. Many of the men writhed in agony, nearly all those able to communicate complained of headache, as if someone were hammering a wedge into their skulls just behind the eyes, and body aches so intense they felt like bones breaking. A few were vomiting. Finally the skin of some of the sailors had changed color. Some showed just a tinge of blue around their lips for fingertips, a few looked almost black."[5]

The Eclectic physicians gave similar descriptions of the 1918 flu: "We were shocked in early October, 1918 when so many of our friends were suddenly attacked by a grave disease with many dying before we could scarcely realize what was in front of us. Course of the disease: A weak, languid, tired aching feeling for 24 hours preceding the chill. The chill lasts from 2-4 hours followed with high fever (99 to 105 degrees), intense headache and severe pain in the lumbar region. ...The first fever extends from 3-5 days and declines for 1-2 days. The patient seems to convalesce for 1-2 days then the second fever presents with the same severity lasting 1-3 days. It is during this phase the patient is apt to contract pneumonia or a congested lung. Hemorrhage from the nose, throat and lungs is very frequent with a severe, harsh cough with an intense heaviness and weighty feeling over the lungs."[6]

One physician reported that the first wave of the epidemic ended in June but reappeared in early October in a more virulent form. Nearly every case presented with pulmonary symptoms to some degree and was serious in about one out of four. The pulmonary complications included bronchitis, pleurisy, broncho-pneumonia and lobar pneumonia and edema of the lungs. Other complications were rare but there were cases of nephritis and one of purulent meningitis.[7]

Symptoms varied in different parts of the country: "The current epidemic symptoms are sudden discomfort, severe headache, mostly frontal, muscular pains in the loins extending to the extremities, marked weakness, suddenly elevated temperature, frequently with chilly sensations, a marked redness of face and eyes with a general feeling of intense heat. Sclera assumes a yellowish appearance, sometimes there is an icteric hue over the whole body. The pharyngeal and nasal membranes are inflamed causing severe pain in the frontal sinuses and at time aphonia from involvement of the larynx. In this part of the country we have an enteric form of the disease that is a little longer in duration and often mistaken for typhoid."[8]

Physicians reported that the pneumonia that followed the 1918 influenza had some unusual aspects. "Catarrhal or lobular pneumonia seemed to predominate, especially in the younger patients. The pneumonia developed about the third or fourth day of the influenza and more often after the temperature had subsided from the initial disease. The temperature ran very high, sometimes as high as 105 and remained so for from one to five days. . . . The expectorated mucus was white and frothy with occasional streaks of blood; in the majority of cases it was very scanty. Digestion was much more disturbed than in ordinary pneumonia. There was constipation. The tongue was coated with a dirty white coat, the breath was very offensive and smelled more like the breath found in septic peritonitis or typhoid fever."[9]

"The sudiferous glands were very active, excreting a foul smelling mucus that very much resembled the odor of measles. The nervous system was greatly disturbed. Most cases presented delirium and the general nervous system was excited to the extent of producing a quiver over the whole body. Ausculation would show a complete absence of the vesicular sounds over a considerable portion of the lung while the percussion would be resonant. Unlike the usual course of pneumonia, the symptoms were more severe while they lasted but in most cases were of shorter duration."[10]

Avian Influenza (H5N1) Symptoms

In 2006, attention was focused on avian influenza, or "Bird Flu," as the strain that might give rise to the next pandemic. Its symptoms were somewhat different from those of the 1918 influenza. The initial symptoms of avian influenza include a high fever, and influenza-like symptoms (fever, cough, sore throat, muscle aches). Diarrhea, vomiting, abdominal pain, chest pain, and bleeding from the nose and gums have also been reported as early symptoms in some patients. Watery diarrhea without blood appears to be fairly common, and not all confirmed patients have respiratory symptoms. In two patients from southern Vietnam, the clinical diagnosis was acute encephalitis; neither patient had respiratory symptoms when first examined. In a case from Thailand, the patient had fever and diarrhea, but no respiratory symptoms.[11]

In most, breathing difficulties tended to develop about five days after the first symptoms. Respiratory distress, a hoarse voice, and a crackling sound when inhaling are common. Sputum production is variable and sometimes bloody. Almost all patients develop pneumonia. During the Hong Kong avian flu outbreak, all severely ill patients had primary viral pneumonia, which, of course, did not respond to antibiotics. In patients infected with avian influenza, deterioration is rapid. In severe cases, clinicians have observed respiratory failure three to five days after symptom onset. Another common feature is multi-organ dysfunction.[12] Avian flu appears to be most dangerous to younger children but has also killed young adults.

Is H5N1 Likely To Be The Next Pandemic Flu?

Because regular contact with backyard chicken flocks is common in Asia, the few reported cases of bird flu arise out what may be hundreds of thousands of human exposures. Avian flu is probably underreported because people may not realize they have it, but the facts strongly indicate that avian flu is not tending to spread in the human population to any particular degree even after more than seven years of opportunity to mutate and spread.

Of course, it is still possible that H5N1 will mutate into a deadly strain of human influenza, and the virus has mutated to a more virulent form in recent years, affecting large numbers of animals. Before the outbreaks continued cropping up, most researchers predicted that the next pandemic would be an H2 strain but many experts now think H5N1 may be "the one." Many other experts think not. "There are many other more likely candidates," they say. The experts do agree that pandemics will continue to occur in the future, as they have in the past, and that we must be prepared for the next one. Our inability to know what type of flu will spread makes vaccine preparation nearly impossible.

Conventional Treatments for Pandemic Influenza

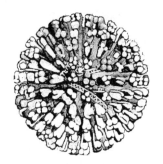

Vaccines

A vaccine essentially teaches our immune system to recognize characteristic aspects of an intruder. Small amounts of a dead virus are injected, allowing the immune system to become familiar with the virus without mobilizing a strong immune response. This familiarity allows the person to quickly mount an effective attack when a live virus with the same or nearly identical signal components intrudes.

Most flu vaccines are produced by injecting a live flu virus into fertilized chicken eggs where the virus replicates. The virus in the eggs is then killed with chemicals, extracted and the dead virus is used as the vaccine. However, some viral strains rapidly kill fertilized chicken eggs making it very difficult to quickly produce large amounts of vaccine. Both the avian and the 1918 flu pose this problem. There are ways around this problem but creating a vaccine for a recently mutated and lethal flu strain will take many months during which time the virus can continue to infect humans.

An additional problem in vaccine production is keeping a sufficient number of laying hens alive in the presence of a flu strain that kills them within hours of exposure. "Vaccine hens" are housed in a sterile environment but the challenge of keeping millions of them laying healthy eggs and keeping vaccine workers healthy while they handle the eggs in a pandemic lethal to chickens, eggs, and humans is troubling. It will take about one chicken egg per person -- plus six months time -- to create a vaccine the traditional way. At last count, there were 297 million people in the US and 6.4 billion people in the world.

Work is also underway to create a nasal spray vaccine that contains live, weakened viruses instead of the traditional vaccine. However, production of spray vaccines also requires eggs. It is, of course, frightening to distribute a live, highly infectious and potentially lethal spray without lengthy testing to ensure that it is sufficiently "weakened" not to cause the disease it is supposed to prevent. Research is also ongoing to manufacture vaccines in cell cultures. Cancerous cells from animals are used because they grow quickly and live long. However, vaccines manufactured from cancer cells have not yet been approved in part because of concern that the vaccine may include some unknown cancer-causing factor.

Society is investing heavily in vaccines in the hope that they will be available to provide some protection against a mutated pandemic flu but no one is certain that effective vaccines will be available. Of course, the *degree* of effectiveness is critical because vaccines are not entirely safe.

Back in 1976, the world feared a different flu pandemic, the Swine Flu. Forty million people were inoculated with a vaccine made in haste after a single army recruit died of what was designated the new lethal flu. The epidemic never emerged and vaccinations were halted because many who were inoculated were struck with paralyzing Guillain-Barre syndrome.[13] In Guillain-Barre, the body attacks the nervous system, leading to pain, muscle weakness or paralysis for which there is no cure. Additionally (and possibly related) many flu vaccines contain thimerosal, a compound that is 49.6 percent mercury by weight. This is troubling as the flu shot given many babies today can contain 12.5 micrograms of mercury, and a baby "should" weigh 275 pounds for a vaccine containing that amount of mercury to be considered safe according to the Environmental Protection Agency standards.[14] In addition, vaccine makers often add aluminum hydroxide to boost the immune response to the vaccine. Aluminum may or may not be a causative factor in Alzheimer's disease; it is in any event not considered a healthful mineral.

Tamiflu® And Other Antiviral Drugs

Viruses use their neuramidase (the "N" in H5N1) to prevent the viral particles from clumping together when they burst out of their host cell. Tamiflu® and Relenza® are drugs that inhibit neuramidase. Amantadine® and Rimantadine®, two other antiviral drugs, target a different viral spike, M2. Unfortunately, the flu virus is usually able to become resistant to the M2 drugs, often within two or three days. The H5 viruses currently circulating in Southeast Asia are already resistant to M2 drugs as are most influenza strains circulating in the United States.

Most governments have been stockpiling Tamiflu, and many consumers are hoarding the drug as well. The government thinks a human outbreak may be contained by "blanketing" communities where an outbreak occurs with Tamiflu to reduce the severity of the disease, protect healthy people, and prevent it from spreading. Recently, the government also placed multi-million dollar orders for Relenza and is encouraging states to stockpile that drug as well.

How Effective And Safe Are Antiviral Drugs?

Tamiflu reduced the severity and duration of usual influenza strains when taken within 48 hours of the onset of symptoms. It somewhat protects caregivers from getting the flu. However, the studies are small and the data is limited. In seven confirmed bird flu victims treated with Tamiflu, two survived and five died. Some attribute this failure to the fact that the drug needs to be given so early in the disease progression. The two avian flu victims who survived got the drug sooner (within four to five days from onset of symptoms) and got a complete 5-day course. The five who died were given Tamiflu on average from the ninth day. It is possible the results would have been better had they gotten the Tamiflu earlier but we do not know if timing was critical. Ultimately, we do not know if Tamiflu will work in a virulent pandemic influenza.

Moreover, a young Vietnamese girl with bird flu was found to have a Tamiflu-resistant strain. This suggests that the avian flu may rapidly become resistant to the drug. Recent animal studies suggest that avian flu is less susceptible to Tamiflu than when the virus first appeared in 1997. Mice infected with a 2004 strain of the virus needed a higher dose and longer treatment with Tamiflu than the mice infected with the 1997 strain but the drug was still effective. Mice studies show that a standard five-day course protected only 50% of the mice infected with H5N1 but survival rose to 80% when they got the drug for eight days. In the test tube, H3N2 and H1N1 strains developed resistance to Tamiflu. This means that our antiviral drugs may ultimately not be very helpful in a pandemic, especially if they are widely used.

Side effects from antiviral drugs are usually mild. Tamiflu may cause dizziness, jitters, and insomnia. The Japanese government added a warning of psychosis to Tamiflu's label after two teenagers on the drug committed suicide. There have been 48 reports of psychiatric side effects associated with Tamiflu use in Europe but medical authorities are not sure they were drug related as the flu and high fever also can cause hallucinations.

Seldom mentioned is the fact that the drug approval research on Tamiflu showed that it causes bone deformities in rabbits and rats exposed to the drug in utero.[15] It is therefore contraindicated in pregnancy. Tamiflu is also metabolized poorly by young infants who may, as a result, be exposed to ten times the amount of its toxic compounds than adults. Thus, Tamiflu is not recommended for infants less than a year old. It is also secreted in the breast milk and should not be taken by women who are nursing babies. There has been no discussion about how Tamiflu can be used effectively in a pandemic if it cannot safely be given to pregnant and lactating women, and young children. Tamiflu also caused osteomalacia (a painful, softening of the bones or rickets) in some laboratory animals. The Federal Drug Administration accepted the manufacturer's opinion that this was due to inherent defects in the animals, and further investigations into this side effect were not requested.[16]

The other neuramidase inhibitor on the market, Relenza, has a yet sketchier profile. The FDA initially refused to approve it because Relenza provided minimal benefits to healthy adults in clinical trials, and actually worsened the outcome for "high risk" groups such as the elderly, and those with respiratory and cardiac ailments.[17] It is not approved for prophylactic use, that is to prevent caregivers from getting the flu, and it is not approved for children under the age of seven. It has a relatively good safety profile except that it appears to have a tendency to cause bronchospasms, and has caused fatal bronchospasms.

Another problem is that Relenza caused lymphoma in laboratory animals. This was noted in the approval process but as the drug was intended for short term use (two doses every 12 hours for five days), the consensus was that this presented a minimal risk to users. Officials, however, noted that this issue would have to be revisited if Relenza were to be prescribed as a prophylactic over a longer period. Of course, at present there is no reliable data showing that Relenza is effective as a preventative. Additional problems include that the flu virus developed resistance to the drug in the test tube as well as in one patient in the pre-approval testing, and that it is a difficult drug to administer. Relenza is given intranasally, and in the studies many patients had a hard time learning how to use the drug properly. There is real concern that patients sick with a virulent flu strain will not be able to learn how to use the drug quickly enough. And time is of the essence: any benefit from Relenza requires that it be taken within 48 hours of the first flu symptoms.

One of the most important planned uses for the stockpiled antiviral drugs is to protect caregivers and other important personnel from getting influenza. But, in order to prevent influenza, these drugs must be taken continuously, and the virus must not develop resistance to the drug as it moves through large numbers of people taking the drugs. Many flu pandemics, including the 1918 pandemic, lasted a full year. Taking Tamiflu or Relenza as protection during such a prolonged pandemic is not feasible. And, as a practical matter, most Americans are not going to have access to enough Tamiflu or Relenza to see them through even a short illness, if they have access to any at all.

Scary Responses To The Threat Of A Pandemic

Enormous research efforts are being funded with the goal of preventing the next influenza pandemic. Some of this research is actually more disturbing than the H5N1 virus because the research itself may ignite a devastating pandemic.

Researchers have recreated the 1918 flu virus, and infected mice with it. This virus is extremely virulent. In four days it generated 39,000 times more virus particles in the animals' lungs than a modern flu strain did. All the mice died within six days. The lead researcher commented: "I did not expect it to be so lethal." This work was done in an enhanced biosafety Level 3 laboratory. A bacteriologist commented that the work should have been done in a Level 4 lab because of the significant risk that the virus would accidentally escape into the environment. He pointed out that a SARS virus accidentally escaped from three different Level 3 labs in recent years. The lead researcher countered that Level 3 was safe enough, and added that, even if the virus escaped, people probably have some immunity to it. The recreated 1918 flu virus is now being worked on in other labs in various parts of the world.

Researchers at the United States Centers for Disease Control (CDC) are combining the H5N1 strain with the human H3N2 influenza strain "under tight security." In the fall of 2006, the CDC will test the 254 new influenza combinations they created in live animals to determine how infectious they are.[18] Their research is highly controversial because of the potential for bioterrorism. It is also disturbing because escapes from labs happen, and because humans do make mistakes: Three mice carrying a deadly plague strain recently disappeared from a New Jersey lab. Health officials downplayed the health risk assuring that the mice probably died quickly – and, we hope, did not have any fleas.

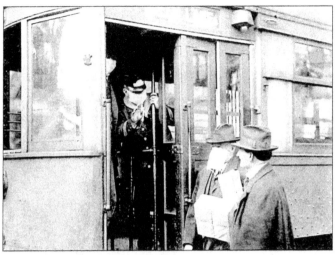

Trolley conductor prevents passenger without mask from boarding (1918).

Our Plan For The Pandemic

The current Bush administration has a multi-billion dollar plan to combat the flu.[19] The plan includes measures like closing airports, imposing snow days on schools to prevent children from spreading the disease, and forcing patients to wear masks. If properly used, face masks do prevent a person from spreading influenza. However, it is hard to visualize how patients coughing up phlegm, suffocating in effusions, and taking antiviral drugs will be able to comply. As for the general public, masks may not provide complete protection from the flu as many avian flu strains are also absorbed through the eyes. Masks also collect the virus on their surface, and unless carefully used and disposed of, can actually spread the disease. Most masks and other protective equipment lose their barrier properties if washed, and cannot be reused.[20] This means that we would need an enormous number of masks in a year long pandemic.

The plan also includes rationing of antiviral drugs and ventilators, and having the army enforce quarantines or control riots. President Bush's plan to invoke the power to declare martial law and use the army to quarantine citizens and prevent riots is a somewhat frightening prospect. First, the 1918 flu was in large measure spread by the military. The military often live in close quarters (somewhat reminiscent of poultry farms) and can provide a very good breeding ground for a virus. And even if the soldiers themselves are somewhat protected by vaccines or Tamiflu, they may continue to be able to infect the populace. (See chapter How Are The Chickens Doing?). And as soldiers are deployed to quarantine the population, then deployed to another location, or allowed to return to their homes, they may become the vector for the flu.

Second, the pandemic may not be immediately at hand. It may be years before it arrives. The government thought swine flu was imminent when one young soldier died. There are few safeguards in place to determine how and when the politicians may decide to declare an epidemic, shut down travel, and quarantine large groups of people.

Finally, the plan includes massive expenditures on antiviral drugs and vaccines. The Department of Health and Human Services is investing $165 million to build a stockpile of 20 million doses of an experimental H5N1 vaccine without any evidence that the vaccine will work if the virus jumps to humans. US public health officials plan to buy 44 million doses of primarily Tamiflu, and are encouraging the state government to buy another 31 million doses. The Pentagon ordered $58 million worth for US troops around the world, and we may ultimately spend over a billion dollars on Tamiflu.

Every Cloud Has a Silver Lining

Our purchases of antiviral drugs and vaccines have some interesting economic effects, particularly because there is doubt that these treatments will work in a pandemic. Each Tamiflu pill retails for about $8 so it could cost as much as $160 million just to treat 200,000 people. To blunt a pandemic, a much larger number of people would have to be treated. Many experts think that one-third to one-half of the population would need to take the drug. This translates into 100 million Americans taking Tamiflu daily for some length of time, or billions of doses. We will be spending an enormous amount of money for a drug that may have limited effectiveness to begin with, and that the virus may quickly develop resistance to.

So where is the silver lining? Tamiflu was created by Gilead Sciences, a California company, and was licensed to the Swiss manufacturer Roche Holding AG in 1996. Sales of Tamiflu reached $1.2 billion in 2005, a figure that could triple next year as governments and private purchasers scramble to fill their planned antiviral stockpiles.[21] Roche pays Gilead royalties of between 14 percent and 22 percent. Interestingly, Donald Rumsfeld, until he resigned and joined the Bush administration, was the chairman of Gilead. He did recuse himself from any decisions involving Gilead when he became Secretary of Defense in early 2001 but his shares are valued at between $5 and $25 million, and growing. Other Gilead board members include former Secretary of State George Shultz, who made about $7 million from stock sales in 2005. The wife of former Republican governor Pete Wilson is also on Gilead's board. Thus, Gilead may be the biotech company with the ultimate political connections. Relenza, manufactured by Glaxo Wellcome, has made fewer sales but in the last six months of 2005, the French, Australian and German governments ordered 12.5 million doses of Relenza. Before 2005, Glaxo Wellcome sold about 500,000 doses a year. [22]

Vaccine and other antiviral drug research is also booming, and the government is being pressured into helping make vaccines more profitable. A fellow of the Hoover Institute, an influential conservative think-tank, recently recommended that the government should fund research on vaccine production techniques and cross-subtype vaccines, guarantee purchases of approved vaccines, and indemnify vaccine manufacturers against liability for any harm caused by their vaccines in order to make the industry more profitable. [23] Congress in 2004 added influenza vaccine to the Vaccine Injury Compensation Program that gives vaccine manufacturers broad liability protection for injuries caused by their products. [24] Notwithstanding, Republicans continue to introduce bills that would make it almost impossible to sue for harm caused by a vaccine, antiviral drug or other "pandemic or epidemic product" used during an influenza pandemic. [25]

Influenza and Pregnancy

Pregnant woman are more vulnerable to influenza than any other group. The death rate for pregnant women hospitalized with influenza in the 1918 pandemic ranged from 23 to 71 percent. Of the women who survived, 26 percent lost their child. [26] Influenza has been connected with miscarriage and death of pregnant women as far back in time as 1557.

The preparedness plans do not provide many answers, if

any, for pregnant women. The available antiviral drugs have not been studied in pregnant women, and may not be safe in pregnancy. Studies submitted to the FDA showed that Tamiflu caused bone deformities in rabbit and rat offspring. Unfortunately, this aspect of Tamiflu has not been researched beyond that done to support its approval by the FDA. Instead of asking for more research, the FDA approved Tamiflu with labeling restrictions that state that it "should be used in pregnancy only if the potential benefit justifies the potential risk to the fetus." The same instructions apply to its use during lactation. Of course, because Tamiflu is not safe for pregnant women, pregnant women are not included in clinical studies on its efficacy as a prophylactic. This makes it difficult to decide if its potential benefit in a pandemic outweighs its risk of birth defects.

How Are The Chickens Doing?

One way to measure the effectiveness of the currently proposed plans for prevention, drugs, and vaccines is to examine how the chickens are faring in their pandemic. So far, they are not doing well at all.

The first outbreak of bird flu occurred in Hong Kong in 1997. All poultry in the territory were culled. Markets selling live poultry were strictly regulated with monthly off-days when the markets were emptied and cleaned. New outbreaks continue to occur in Hong Kong and elsewhere in Asia despite such "intensive control measures."

Outbreaks and chicken deaths continue even though chickens in China have been "blanketed" with an estimated

2.6 billion doses of the antiviral drug Amantadine since early 2004. Hundreds of millions of birds have been culled or killed to stop the spread of the virus, sometimes in rather gruesome ways such as the thousands of chickens that were buried alive.

Veterinary experts are divided on the wisdom of poultry vaccination, as it appears that the vaccines do not completely protect birds from dying, and vaccines do not completely prevent the virus from replicating, shedding, and spreading. Milder cases of flu sometimes cause only ruffled feathers and a drop in egg production that may go unnoticed but may nonetheless be able to infect the people who handle the birds.

Not only may vaccinations not protect chickens from the virus, they can on occasion worsen the situation. A poultry outbreak in Japan was caused by the use of a vaccine with a live H5N2 virus -- post-production testing of the vaccine failed to ensure that the virus was dead. Japan had another similar event in 2004 when an outbreak of classical swine fever was caused by an unauthorized vaccine. Fake bird flu vaccines for poultry were found in China at the site of a recent outbreak.

Ultimately, more than seven years work on limiting the spread of a known strain of influenza in poultry has not eliminated the epidemic that continues to infect and kill birds. The government intends to use similar measures to protect us in a human pandemic but without a vaccine targeted at a known strain of influenza (remember, the virus will have to mutate to cause a pandemic). If these measures do not work in chickens, what reason do we have to believe that they will be effective in humans?

Herbal Remedies for Influenza

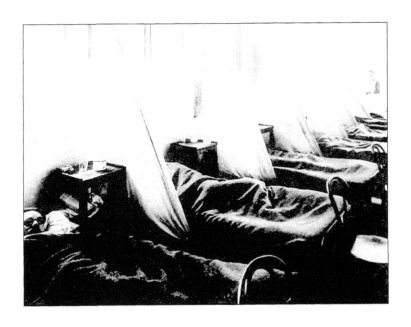

Given our present inability to respond effectively to a pandemic, it makes tremendous sense to investigate the plant remedies physicians reported were used successfully in the very worst pandemic known. However, while mind-boggling amounts of money are being spent on drugs with questionable effectiveness, at least in this country, no money is being spent on research on herbal treatments for influenza.

This is not a new problem. Most herbal remedies are poorly researched because, until very recently, herbal medicine studies simply were not funded. Almost all of the existing clinical and pharmacological research on such treatments was done outside the United States. Today, slightly more funding is available, but most research is geared toward finding plant compounds that can be transformed into patentable drugs. There are very few studies trying to learn whether whole plant remedies work. It is not unusual to find a preliminary study showing that the whole plant is more effective in animals than the plant's isolated constituents. Nonetheless, the subsequent studies examine only the isolated constituents. Moreover, people trained in botanical medicine are not invited to participate in the few clinical studies that are done. As a result, the dose and other factors usually do not reflect how the plants should be used, and often do not provide useful clinical information.

Not surprisingly, only a very few of the plants used to treat influenza in 1918 have been studied at all. There is some safety data on a few of them but efficacy data is wholly lacking. As a result, there is no solid information to help an individual decide whether or not to use some or all of them in a pandemic. Some people are comfortable relying on historical evidence of use. Others are uncomfortable using remedies that do not have validated safety studies or proven efficacy. Both positions are reasonable. In a pandemic, each individual will have to weigh their choices and act accordingly. This book does not, and cannot, advocate any particular course of action except to urge that society might benefit greatly if proper efficacy studies into these plants were funded now.

Information Sources on Eclectic Influenza Remedies

Evidence on the effectiveness of herbal treatments of pandemic influenza comes from the texts and articles compiled by a group of physicians known as the "Eclectics." They include articles published in Eclectic medical journals between 1870 and 1930, a survey of over 200 physicians who provided information on their most effective treatments, and a study conducted at an allied military hospital in France.

Why has this information been completely ignored until now? Beginning in the 1700s, the Eclectics and allopathic (or "Regular") physicians battled with each other over how to best treat patients. The outcome of these battles set the stage for modern medicine and led to the current marginalization and fear of herbal medicine. We need to understand these conflicts if we are to understand why society has overlooked highly useful influenza remedies.

Who Were The Eclectics?

The Eclectics were medical doctors who primarily used herbs and natural principles of healing to treat their patients. They were a strong force in American medicine from the 1830s to the early 1900s but disappeared by the 1930s. Their views were shaped in reaction to the "heroic" medicine practiced by the typical allopathic or "Regular" physicians in Europe and the US.

George Washington provides an example of mainstream medicine at that time: On Friday, December 13th, 1799,

George Washington awoke with a painful sore throat, labored breathing, and a fever. He had been soaked by rain the day before. He called for a bleeder who took 12 or 14 ounces of blood from his arm. Washington felt worse the next day and called for his doctors. They prescribed two more bleedings along with two doses of mercury and a cathartic enema. He grew worse. After some debate, his doctors decided to bleed another 32 ounces while giving him a much larger dose of mercury along with a dose of another strong poison, antimony. Blisters were raised on his throat and the soles of his feet. Less than 48 hours after awakening with infected tonsils, George Washington was dead.[27]

This was accepted medical treatment; it had been for centuries and continued to be well into the 1800s. Dr. Benjamin Rush, one of the signers of the Declaration of Independence, taught medicine and advocated bloodletting for almost all conditions. He recommended drawing up to 140 ounces to cure pneumonia. He taught his medical students that mercury was "a safe and nearly universal medicine."[28]

A group of physicians dissatisfied with this aggressive treatment embarked on a different course. They called themselves "Eclectics" from the Greek word for 'select'. Their goal was to find the best remedy for the individual patient, and they chose carefully among different traditions, including those of the homeopaths and the Native Americans. Their primary medicines were herbs, and they believed strongly in nourishing the individual rather than using bleeding, mercury, antimony, and cathartics. They had a strong influence on allopathic medicine, reducing but not eliminating their drastic treatments. Thus, by 1918, Regular physicians no longer prescribed bleedings but they continued to use mercury and strong laxative purges. They continued to favor near toxic doses of plants as well as newly introduced chemicals.

The Eclectics collected information on the use of plants in a wide variety of diseases. They published their own medical journals, and opened medical schools. Their views were liberal, and both women and African Americans graduated from Eclectic medical schools. John Uri Lloyd, a famous pharmacist, joined the Eclectics and zeroed in on plant extraction, working to create medicines that retained the actions of the whole plant. Many tinctures are still made according to his recommendations.

The Eclectics -- as do modern herbalists -- sometimes struggled with the gentleness of their medicines compared to the strength of allopathic drugs. One Eclectic lamented: "Some people will take a few doses of medicine from an Eclectic, and if it don't cure at once, they think there is nothing in it. But they will take large doses of strong drugs week after week, and though they do not improve, they think it is all right because the medicine has a big bulk and a powerful taste. They think it is doing something. Well, so do we. It oftentimes gives the undertaker a job."[29]

Another Eclectic commented that herbal medicines ultimately cured more quickly because "owing to drug complications, it many times takes [allopathic] patients as long to recover from their treatment as it does from the disease." The Eclectics cited statistics to support their claims. Data from public hospitals showed that the 41% of pneumonia patients treated by "Regulars" died compared to a 16% death rate for Eclectic patients. Overall for all diseases, the death rate for Regulars was 6.3% compared to a 4.2% death rate for Eclectics.[30]

So, why are most people unfamiliar with the Eclectics? In large measure, it is the result of the battle the American Medical Association (AMA) waged against them and homeopathic physicians in the early 1900s. The public was left with the strong impression that plant medicines were ineffective and dangerous, and that disease was never treated successfully before the advent of modern drugs.

The Demise Of The Eclectics

Less than a hundred years ago, herbalist Michael Moore explained, we had a rich and diverse community of physicians that represented several sophisticated medical views. These included Regulars, Eclectics, Homeopathists, Chiropractors, and Osteopaths. They went to different medical schools but sat for the same Boards before entering practice. In 1915, there were 155 medical schools of which eight were Eclectic, 15 Homeopathic schools, one Physiomedical, eight Osteopathic, seven African-American only, three women-only. By 1940, the allopathic schools dominated, and the Eclectic schools were gone.[31] This dramatic change was brought about by the "Flexner Report" on the state of medical education in the United States. Today, the report is still praised as having taken the medical curriculum "out of the hands of quacks and put it on a sound scientific footing."[32] But this praise might not continue if more people were aware that the AMA shaped the report to decimate non-Regular medical schools and the public image of non-Regular MDs.

In the 1800s, physician incomes were on par with those of mechanics. The AMA was formed in 1847 and one of its primary goals was to increase the status and the income of Regular physicians. From the beginning the AMA sought to achieve its goals by denouncing the "quackery" of its colleagues, eliminating "alternative" medical schools, and reducing the number of graduating physicians.[33] In 1904, the AMA adopted a plan to close half of the medical schools in the United States. The next year, it formed a Council to "fight the war on quack patent medicines and nostrum trade." But by 1908, the AMA was losing ground due to in-fighting and a lack of money to wage attacks on its colleagues.[34]

This changed when, in 1910, the Carnegie Foundation offered to prepare what is now known as the Flexner Report. The report was "guided very largely" by the AMA but the Carnegie Foundation promised *not* to disclose the AMA's role so the report would have the "weight of a disinterested body, which would then be published far and wide. It would do much to develop public opinion." The Foundation promised the AMA that when "our report comes out it is going to be ammunition in your hands" and urged that it "is desirable, therefore, to maintain in the meantime a position which does not intimate an immediate connection between our two efforts."[35]

Having struck this deal, the Carnegie Foundation hired Abraham Flexner, an unemployed schoolmaster, to prepare a report on the state of medical education in America. Flexner was not a physician, and had no background in the clinical care of patients. Nonetheless, he was chosen to examine and critique each of the 155 American medical schools. On average, he spent less than a day actually inspecting the various schools. Flexner often sought the advice of the AMA, and his brother, Simon Flexner, an MD and director of the Rockefeller Institute for Medical Research.

The publication of the Flexner Report created headlines in newspapers across America. Although many medical journals criticized it as full of errors, "raw malice, and unpercolated venom," Flexner's descriptions of inadequate, filthy medical schools filled with decaying cadavers grabbed the headlines and its images swayed the public. The report wanted the supply of doctors reduced so that existing physicians "could make a competent livelihood." Medical schools were to be closed so that only 31 of the 155 schools remained to dramatically reduce the output of new physicians.

The 1910 Flexner Report, true to the AMA view, described chiropractors as "unconscionable quacks" and the Eclectic physicians – who used herbs in the days when allopaths used mercury – as "drug mad." The report recommended closing the three women's schools because women "show a decreasing inclination to enter the profession". Five of the seven African-American medical schools were closed. The report suggested that two remain open because African Americans were a "potential source of infection and contagion" and needed their own physicians. However, hygiene, rather than surgery, was to be accentuated at these two schools. Overall, the report put research before practice. Teachers were to be scientists not clinicians.[36] In 1913, Abraham Flexner, the formerly unemployed schoolmaster, secured a $1.5 million gift from the Carnegie Foundation to Johns Hopkins University and soon thereafter joined the board of Johns Hopkins University to help disperse millions of dollars in grants to develop a chemically-oriented medicine.[37]

Flexner and the AMA raised some valid issues as physician education was often seriously lacking at that time. But their emphasis on the business of medicine, and the foisting of a homogenous, drug- and business-oriented medical model on the public at the expense of diversity in clinical practice was ultimately harmful. Painting alternative medicine as useless quackery has not served the public well. Americans would be healthier if the medical system had remained eclectic – that is, always looking for the best solution for the individual patient, even if that solution is a non-patentable plant medicine.

The Eclectic Legacy

By the 1920s the Eclectic schools were in steep decline and Eclectic physicians were ignored and marginalized by mainstream allopathic medicine. The success the Eclectics had in treating victims of the 1918 influenza pandemic was not brought to the public's attention. While the Eclectics continued to publish in their own journals, their work was ignored by mainstream medicine. Fortunately, a few libraries retained copies of their publications for posterity. This book describes the Eclectic treatment of influenza as reported in three primary sources.

First, Eclectic texts (known as materia medica) remain in print from the Eclectic Institute in Sandy, Oregon. These texts list all of the plant remedies, as well as a few non-herbal remedies, in use at the time of the 1918 pandemic. The texts also describe how to prepare, dose, and administer the herbs.

Second, numerous articles with the word "influenza" in the title were published in the Eclectic Medical Journal between 1873 through 1929, and these articles are accessible through the National Library of Medicine. Medical journal articles at that time were quite different from scientific articles today. Most of the articles were only a few paragraphs long, and typically simply described a case history or experience of a physician. The articles are anecdotal and unconcerned with many details and procedures that we now expect from a scientific study.

Third, there is an extensive amount of information gathered in a survey sent to physicians who purchased plant remedies from Lloyd Brothers. The survey asked what remedies were used to treat influenza and pneumonia during the 1918 pandemic. Lloyd Brothers published the brief responses submitted by 237 physicians.

The Lloyd Brothers' Survey

John Uri Lloyd was a pharmacist, researcher, manufacturer, and author. He had a lifelong professional association with the Eclectics, and worked with them to develop better botanical extracts. He was highly respected by traditional pharmacists as well and was elected president of the American Pharmaceutical Association in 1887. He was awarded three Ebert Prizes for original research, and the Remington Medal, American pharmacy's highest honor, in 1920. He and his brothers owned Lloyd Brothers, a company that manufactured and distributed botanical extracts.

On January 1, 1919, Lloyd Brothers sent a survey to physicians who had purchased their botanical products asking them to reply to five questions:

1. Name six remedies that you consider essential in the treatment of influenza.

2. Name the one you consider to be most important.

3. Name the remedies you consider necessary in treatment of pneumonia.

4. Do you use an application to the chest? If so, what do you employ?

5. Do you practice according to principles of Specific Medication?

The pandemic, although waning, was still active in early 1919. Lloyd Brothers decided that the answers they received were of such great interest to physicians that they decided to publish them immediately. The responses were compiled in the order received and no responses were excluded.

Question number five asked the physicians if they followed the principles of "Specific Medication." Specific Medicine (or Specific Medication) was a core concept in Eclectic medicine. Eclectic physicians focused on their patients' symptoms and prescribed remedies to relieve their specific symptoms rather than working strictly from a diagnois of a disease. In pandemic influenza, symptoms varied greatly from patient to patient. As a result, Eclectic influenza patients might receive very different prescriptions, depending on their symptoms. This approach contrasts sharply with allopathic medicine which first diagnoses the disease and then selects a remedy that is considered appropriate for all patients with that disease.

Most of the surveyed physicians (157) did practice specific medicine but eleven were allopaths, four were homeopathic practitioners, and 65 did not answer the question. And, even among those who said they were Eclectic, some used drugs like calomel (mercury), caffeine, and cathartics, indicating that they used a more allopathic treatment approach. In analyzing the survey for this book, the eleven allopaths and the four homeopaths were excluded, leaving 222 responses. (Appendix B sets out all of the remedies these physicians used to treat influenza.)

Question four asked for the remedies that were necessary for the treatment of pneumonia. Most physicians appeared to respond this question with information on how they treated influenza that caused pulmonary complications but this could not be ascertained with certainty. For instance, one physician noted: "I am in a pneumonia climate, and treat on an average from fifty to a hundred cases annually." While mentioned in the context of individual herbs, pneumonia remedies are not included in the compilation in Appendix B.

Did Eclectic Remedies Work?

Our society has a bias against botanical medicine that makes it difficult for many to even consider that physicians could successfully treat pandemic influenza with plants. In his book "*The Great Influenza*", John Barry comments: "Yet a patient's improvement, of course, does not prove that a therapy works. For example, the 1889 edition of the *Merck Manual of Medical Information* recommended one hundred treatments for bronchitis, each one with its fervent believers, yet the current editor of the manual recognizes that 'none of them worked.'" John Barry is right, improvement does not prove that a therapy works. We should, however, ask ourselves how the editor of Merck knows that none of the 1889 therapies (many of which were herbal) worked. There are *no* studies to support this conclusion, and much history and research to contradict it. Modern medicine has simply accepted without analysis or scientific study the view that, before the advent of modern medical education and antibiotics, sheer luck determined who lived and who died. As part of weighing the credibility of this view, we should perhaps ask ourselves why pharmaceutical companies invest large sums of money studying traditional medicines if it has already been proven that they do not work.

As mentioned earlier, data shows that the Eclectics with their herbal remedies often achieved better results than allopathic physicians did. In patients with hospitalized with pneumonia, 41% of patients treated by allopaths died while only 16% of those treated by Eclectics died. [38]   In fact, in treating pneumonia the Eclectics were doing quite well even by today's standards. A 2005 study reports that "Mortality from pneumococcal pneumonia has remained high despite the introduction of antibiotics and improved intensive care medicine. In recent studies, the case-fatality rate for bacteremic pneumococcal pneumonia ranged from 7% to 35%."[39]

It is true, however, that most of the evidence we have on the effectiveness of Eclectic influenza treatments is anecdotal. The Lloyd Brothers' survey provides much information on how physicians across the country actually treated influenza. However, this survey was sent to physicians who bought remedies from the Lloyd Brothers, and we do not know how many of those surveyed failed to respond. Articles on influenza published in the Eclectic Medical Journal, and other Eclectic journals are also anecdotal. However, they span sixty years (1870-1930), many seasons of influenza, and at least two pandemics

In addition, there is one randomized, controlled, and somewhat blind study that shows the Eclectic's favorite influenza remedy worked well on the 1918 influenza strain. At an allied army hospital in France ("the French Hospital study"), an American and a British physician team administered one of eight drugs to groups of 15 patients with influenza, and compared the patients' progress. Three of the drugs were herbs (aconite, belladonna, and gelsemium) while five were remedies more commonly used by allopathic physicians (aspirin, sodium salicylate, arsenic, quinine, and Dover's powder, a mixture of opium and ipecac).[40]

"Those treated with gelsemium improved in a manner far exceeding those given any other treatment. After a few doses their headache and backache were much relieved, the temperature began to fall and the general condition was observably improved." With the exception of belladonna, none of the other drugs appeared to have the slightest effect.

Patient treatment was not based on symptoms. Instead, patients were randomly selected to receive a remedy based on the order in which they were admitted to the hospital. The physicians worked and evaluated the patients independently of each other. However, because "we are well aware of the fallacies of judgment attending the action of remedies," the test was repeated. The second round of results were so striking that the physician-investigators subsequently decided to use gelsemium to treat all patients with influenza. Because belladonna also showed some benefit, it was also added to the gelsemium formula. (See chapter on Gelsemium for the full formula). In summary, treatment of 937 soldiers sick enough to be hospitalized with influenza suffered a mortality rate of 2.77%, a good result in that population group.[41] (In one sector of the Western front, one-third of American soldiers hospitalized with influenza died of the disease.[42]) Except for rare cases of visual disturbances, there were no side effects.

Finally, many physicians responding to the Lloyd Brothers' survey volunteered data on the number of influenza cases they treated as well as the number of deaths they experienced. In a total of 31,198 reported cases, the mortality rate among their flu patients was about 0.6%. In the 1918 pandemic on average at least 2.8% of flu victims died, and that number is considered by many to be a low estimate. Eclectic patients may have suffered fewer fatalities because their physicians prescribed remedies for the *individual* patient's symptoms rather than attempting to treat a disease. This may have been of particular value in the 1918 pandemic because it was a disease that varied greatly in how it expressed itself in different patients. (See chapter on Pandemic Influenza Symptoms.)

In the French Hospital study, the allopathic model was followed. That is, influenza was treated with a set prescription regardless of the specific symptoms of any given patient. The physicians in charge of the study used a formula that combined gelsemium and belladonna. The Eclectics taught that these herbs tended to cancel each other out when combined. "Hence flows the *shot-gun* method of prescribing, whereby the more common drugs are combined in platoons, and fired into the sick ... all kinds of activities represented in the same bottle ... we find the doctor ignoring the law of medicinal incompatibles, and combining his remedies so that one neutralizes the other − *as giving belladonna and gelsemium*...."[43] (Emphasis added.)

Of course, Eclectic treatments were not without failures, and some of the physicians reported on their failures both in the Lloyd Brothers' survey and in articles published in the Eclectic Medical Journal. Overall, however, the information strongly supports the conclusion that even difficult influenza cases were treated successfully by the Eclectics.

The Safety of the Eclectic Remedies

The American Herbal Products Association has published a safety guide that classifies the safety of many botanicals.[44] This information has been included where available. In many instances, however, we have only historical use to guide us because the herbs have not been researched.

Some of the Eclectic remedies are gentle and safe for general use. They have been used to treat influenza for hundreds, if not thousands, of years. Others, however, fall into a category of herbs called low dose herbs. These plants can be used effectively in drop doses but are dangerous when used in larger amounts. A few may cause problems if used inappropriately for the wrong symptoms. They should not be used by an inexperienced person − a person not trained in how to determine if a patient's symptoms match the specific indications the Eclectics described. No one, based on this book, should take it upon themselves to experiment with these herbs. Instead, those interested in having access to these treatments in a pandemic should seek out a practitioner who is trained in their use before the next pandemic strikes.

Herbal Remedies in Pregnancy

We do not know if the Eclectic remedies will affect the unborn child. Many commonly used plants are not recommended for use in pregnancy exactly because safety data is lacking. There is usually no data indicating that they are harmful, they simply have not been studied in pregnancy. Several physicians in the Lloyd Brothers' survey mentioned treating pregnant women. Two physicians in the survey noted that they had each lost a woman patient in her sixth month of pregnancy. But another physician wrote: "I had several cases where women were delivered during the pneumonia of influenza. All were heavily dosed with Echinacea. One woman was delivered with a temperature of 104.5, pulse 130. Consolidation of left lung almost complete – recovery." Yet another said he treated 13 cases of pregnant women with no deaths and no miscarriages. His primary remedy was gelsemium (30 drops in four ounces of water) and a chest application.

Finally, one physician stated that he found veratrum to be the most important herb in pregnant women. As discussed in the chapter on veratrum, it causes severe birth defects in sheep if the ewe eats it during the 14th week of pregnancy but otherwise does not seem to affect baby lambs. We have no idea how it acts in pregnant women.

The Possible Danger of Cytokine Storms

Recently, newspapers reported that the avian flu virus sets off a tremendous immune response, a "cytokine storm," that actually causes the often fatal respiratory complications. People now worry that herbs that stimulate the immune system, such as echinacea, should be avoided in influenza as they may stimulate an already over-reactive system. Research indicates that, to the contrary, herbs appear to quiet these "cytokine storms."

The human immune system consists of billions of cells that use a variety of chemical messengers to keep the system informed and functioning appropriately. These chemical messengers include cytokines and chemokines. There are many different types of cytokines, chemokines, and other immune factors that play a role in fighting off viral infections such as influenza. Viruses, as might be expected, attempt to evade and disarm this system.

The research shows that a virus from a patient who died of avian flu dramatically hyper-induced pro-inflammatory cytokines compared to various strains of seasonal influenza. In particular, the avian flu strain increased the cytokine interleukin-6 and the chemokine interferon-10.[45] The cytokine storm described in news reports was actually a disregulated immune response induced by the virus.

Rhinoviruses, responsible for the common cold, also disregulate the immune system, although to a much lesser extent than influenza viruses do. In fact, the common cold increases the secretion of at least 31 cytokines and chemokines, including interleukin-6 and interferon-10.[46] It is this virus-induced disregulation that causes the unpleasant symptoms of the cold. Echinacea is commonly used as an immune stimulant to treat colds. Millions of users report that it reduces cold symptoms as well as the duration of the cold.

A researcher noted that, if echinacea in fact stimulated the immune system, it would worsen rather than improve cold symptoms. To explore this dilemma, the researcher applied echinacea to both normal cells and cells infected with a cold virus. In healthy cells, echinacea did increase the secretion of cytokines and chemokines. However, in infected cells, echinacea instead reversed or normalized the viral disregulation of the immune messengers, and quieted the "cytokine storm." It brought the amount of interleukin-6 and interferon-10 produced by the infected cells back to normal values.

Researchers have yet to study how herbs affect cells infected with pandemic influenza. However, there is every reason to believe that herbs that have a long history of use to ease influenza symptoms also have the ability to moderate the virus-induced disregulation of the immune system, and are definitely not contraindicated in influenza.

THE ECLECTIC TREATMENT OF INFLUENZA

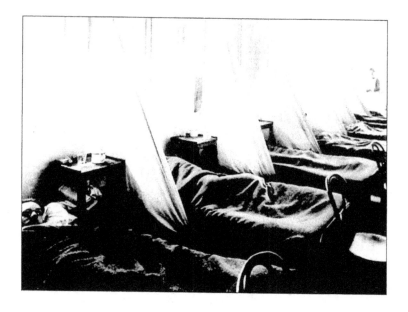

Introduction

The Eclectic remedies are described in this section, more or less in order of importance based on the number of physicians that agreed that the remedy was of great usefulness. The chapter on Honorable Mentions gives a briefer description of an additional twenty plants mentioned in the texts and the survey. This is followed by a chapter that describes a few non-herbal remedies mentioned in the Lloyd Brothers' survey, and a chapter on chest applications. Appendix A is a Glossary that contains definitions of medical and other unusual terms that are mentioned in the text. Appendix B summarizes all of the remedies identified in the Lloyd Brothers' survey. Appendix C is a list of resources for those interested in locating plant remedies or professional practitioners.

An understanding of the type of plant extracts used by the Eclectics will make the discussion of plant remedies more meaningful: The Eclectic doses usually refer to Specific Medicines (sometimes hereafter "SM"). In a work titled *Specific Medication and Specific Medicines*, Dr. John M. Scudder, an Eclectic physician, developed the concept of Specific Medicines.[47] These were usually extracts made from fresh rather than dried herbs. In his book, Scudder explained how physicians could prepare their own Specific Medicines. He typically recommended that seven ounces of herb be macerated (soaked) in 16 ounces of either 76% or 98% alcohol, depending on the plant.

Scudder subsequently sold the rights to use the term "Specific Medicines" to the Lloyd Brothers' company. John Uri Lloyd refined the preparation of these extracts, and produced medicines that were reported to be stronger and clinically more effective than Scudder's original preparations as well as other tincture products available at that time. While we know that Lloyd used special techniques in his manufacturing process, we do not know exactly what his techniques were. His trade secrets remain secret. They may be lost or they may remain locked away as part of the historical files of the pharmaceutical company that ultimately bought Lloyd Brothers. We do know that Lloyd's Specific Medicines usually were extracts prepared from fresh plant material, and probably were made by macerating one part plant in one part of an alcoholic solution, the menstrum.

Given that we no longer have access to Specific Medicines, we do not know with certainty how to translate the Eclectic doses to fit tinctures as they are made today. However, Scudder in his book recommended very similar doses to those that were used for the Lloyd Brothers' Specific Medicines despite the differences in how the two were prepared. Today, many herbalists and manufacturers continue to make fresh plant tinctures much the way Scudder taught. Thus, the Eclectic dosages set out in this book may be accurate. However, it should be noted that many low dose tinctures today are made from dried plant material in much greater dilution than recommended by Scudder or Lloyd. It is possible therefore that the dosages for the stronger Eclectic Specific Medicines are on the low side for some or all of our modern, less concentrated tinctures.

All tinctures have a relatively long shelf life, and, when diluted in water, are easy to administer to a sick patient. Eclectics seldom dispensed herbs as capsules, and the medicinal effects and doses described in this book cannot be assumed to apply to herb capsules. Eclectics occasionally prescribed herbs as teas, and the herb boneset in particular was sometimes used as a diaphoretic tea, but none of the physicians whose comments were reviewed for this book recommended herbs other than in tincture form.

Finally, Scudder also developed and refined the concept of "Specific Indications." The Eclectics based their prescriptions on an assessment of the patient's symptoms rather than on the diagnosis of a disease. When this book summarizes a plant's Specific Indications, it is describing a set of patient symptoms that the Eclectics knew responded to a particular plant remedy.

Biographies

The chapters on Eclectic remedies draw on the work of a number of Eclectic physicians and modern practitioners who were or are respected teachers in the field of botanical medicine. Brief biographies of these individuals are provided for general interest and the sake of clarity.

John Bastyr (1912-1995) was a naturopathic physician and founder of Bastyr University. He had a vast knowledge of medicinal plants, and trained many of the licensed naturopathic physicians in practice today. His teachings have been compiled by Dr. William A. Mitchell, Jr, ND in a book titled *Plant Medicine in Practice*.[48]

Harvey Wickes Felter (1865-1927) was an Eclectic physician and the author of two important Eclectic texts: *The Eclectic Materia Medica, Pharmacology and Therapeutics*[49] and *King's American Dispensatory*[50] which he compiled with John Uri Lloyd. Much of the information on Eclectic treatments comes from these two texts.

David Hoffmann is a British herbalist who practices in North America. He has written several widely used texts on botanical medicine, including *Medical Herbalism, the science and practice of herbal medicine*.[51]

Daniel E Moerman is a professor of anthropology at the University of Michigan. Most of the information on the Native American uses of plants discussed in this book are drawn from Moerman's book *Native American Ethnobotany*.[52]

Michael Moore is an herbalist and director of the Southwest School of Botanical Medicine. He has had a strong influence on herbalism in North America, and has taught many practitioners how to use North American plants. He has an abundance of knowledge on Eclectics, and maintains a website where many of their texts and journals are available. He is the author of many widely used texts on medicinal plants and their uses. Moore's recommended doses for tinctures are provided for most of the remedies discussed in this book.

John M. Scudder (1829-1887) was an Eclectic physician who originated the concepts of Specific Indications and Specific Medicines. He wrote a number of texts, and was a very influential Eclectic.

Rudolf Weiss (1895-1991) was a German physician who used plant remedies in a wide variety of ailments. He continues to influence the practice of many North American botanical prescribers, and his book *Weiss's Herbal Medicine, classic edition*[53] is a widely used botanical textbook.

Eric Yarnell is a naturopathic physician and a professional herbalist. He teaches at Bastyr University and is the author of numerous texts and articles on botanical medicine.

General Eclectic Advice On Treating Influenza

*"Cover up each cough and sneeze,
if you don't you'll spread disease."*[54]

The general advice given influenza patients has not changed much from the time of the Eclectics to the present: Bed rest and plenty of fluids. "The remedies for influenza are few and direct. If the attack is abrupt and there is much pain, give the patient a warm bath, put him to bed and administer hot ginger tea, hot lemonade or similar hot infusion."

The Eclectics often used tepid sponge baths to bring down the fever, and considered it more useful than ice or cold water. A tepid sponge bath was given by constantly sponging the head with warm water, drawing the sponge back and forth and at the same time fanning the person. A modern meta-analysis of the limited clinical trial evidence concluded that tepid sponge baths are effective for reducing fever, at least in children.

In the 1918 pandemic, Eclectics said it was very important that the patient rest, both mentally and physically, and many physicians commented that complications were more common in patients who got up and about too early. Then, as now, working people and those caring for sick family members had a hard time complying with this directive. The Eclectics also noted that sleep was necessary to allow recovery, and that sleeplessness often occurred in the feverish patients and caused complications if not countered. In the French Hospital study, sleep was considered so important that heroin was sometimes administered to ensure that the patient got a good night's sleep. The Ecletics, however, usually relied on herbal sedatives such as *Passiflora incarnata* (passionflower) to help the patient rest.

Most Eclectics were adamant that aspirin and other coal-tar remedies (synthetic medicines) were damaging to the influenza patient. Aspirin can, of course, have serious side effects in children with influenza, and is no longer administered to them. Eclectics felt aspirin weakened the already stressed hearts of patients. They also tended to disapprove of pain medicines that depressed the system, such as codeine, especially where there were pulmonary complications.

Experimental vaccines were available back in 1918. Of course, the viral nature of the disease was not understood at the time, and vaccines and sera were prepared against various bacteria from patients who died of lung complications. These were widely recommended by allopathic physicians, and the following advertisement appeared in the Eclectic Medical Journal: "Dr. E. C. Rosenow of the Mayo Clinic reported on the use of a prophylactic vaccine last winter. There were 100,000 cases under observation, with 300,000 controls. He declared that the incidence of influenza was about three times as common and the death rate five times as high among the uninoculated as among the vaccinated persons. Parke, Davis & Company's Influenza-Pneumonia Vaccine is prepared essentially in accordance with the original formula and method of Dr. Rosenow. It is administered in three injections, at intervals of six or seven days."[55]

Most of the Eclectics warned against the use of vaccines of unknown efficacy, and some suggested that a patient vaccinated and infected with influenza at about the same time seemed to fare poorly. This can happen with some frequency in an epidemic as it usually takes a few weeks for the vaccine to effectively "teach" the immune system to respond to the virus.

Remedies Useful in Seasonal and Pandemic Influenza

The following three remedies, boneset, black cohosh, and pleurisy root, were used by many physicians to treat the 1918 pandemic. They have a long history of use by Native Americans, and remain widely used today. They are considered safe for general use.

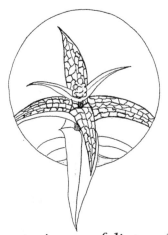

Eupatorium perfoliatum L.
(Boneset, thoroughwort, Indian sage)

The name "boneset" comes from this plant's successful use in influenza pandemics that caused such severe pain that the patients felt like their bones were breaking.

Many Native American tribes used boneset for colds, fever, sore throat, chills, influenza, pneumonia, and pleurisy.

Herbalists, naturopathic physicians, and other modern practitioners continue to use boneset similarly, especially for febrile diseases.

The German physician Dr. Rudolf Weiss explained that boneset is useful in acute viral diseases where antibiotics are ineffective, primarily in influenza, and is believed to enhance resistance to infection. "For obvious reasons it is difficult to get an objective assessment of the anti-infectious effect, but practical experience indicates that it exists, explaining the widespread use of these drugs, particularly as they certainly can do no harm."[56] The above-ground parts of the plant are used, and many practitioners think it is a more effective medicine if tinctured fresh. It is diaphoretic when taken as a hot tea, and the tincture is usually dispensed in hot water to capture this effect.

An early study showed that the plant has antibacterial activity in vitro against *Staphyloccus aureus* and *Escherichia coli*. It contains eupatorin characterized both as a hydroxyflavone (antioxidant) and methoxyflavone (anti-inflammatory).[57] Some of its sesquiterpene lactones and polysaccharide fractions showed immunostimulatory effects in vitro.

The plant belongs to a plant family that often contains liver toxins, pyrrolizidine alkaloids. Although they have not been identified in boneset, it may nonetheless contain them, and should not be used casually.[58] In large doses it can be emetic and cathartic.

Eclectic View Of The Plant

The Eclectics considered boneset a very valuable medicine. "In every epidemic of influenza it has been used with great advantage. During the severe pandemic of 1918-1919 it was one of the safest and most successful remedies employed and contributed much to the successful management of disease under Eclectic treatment." They noted that boneset was also used as a prophylactic but pointed out that its prophylactic action was unproven. However, they also noted: "That cases were rendered milder, deep-seated pain promptly relieved, cough and respiratory irritation lessened, and recovery expedited under the liberal administration of eupatorium is a matter of record. It is especially valuable to relive the intolerable backache and pain in the limbs."

A warm infusion of boneset is diaphoretic and emetic, and is useful in epidemic influenza, in febrile diseases, catarrh and colds with hoarseness and pleuritic pains. In influenza, it relieves pain in the limbs and back. If deep-seated pain is due to a febrile condition, boneset will relieve it. In coughs, it especially helps the elderly and the weak lacking the strength to cough up the abundance of mucus caused by the influenza.

The Eclectics found boneset most useful for patients with a full and large pulse, with the pulse current exhibiting little waves. It was also used if the patient had a full and hot skin that tended to be moist even during the progress of fever or in a patient with a cough, troubled breathing, and pain in the chest. Other indications for use of boneset are influenzal cough and aching pains with turbid urine and frequent urination.

Use In Pandemic Influenza

In 1899, one physician commented that boneset was very valuable in allaying cough with high fever, free perspiration and lack of power to expectorate.[59] In a review of influenza in 1915, a physician recommended boneset any time black cohosh failed to relieve pain.[60] Another physician commented that almost the whole range of influenza symptoms could be controlled with boneset and gelsemium. Boneset is "absolutely safe under all conditions. If too much is used, emesis is the only unpleasant result."[61] In 1918, it was reported "recent experiences point to [boneset] as being one of the best agents to give quick results in epidemic influenza."[62]

Boneset gained popularity as part of a preventative formula after the following announcement was published in 1918: "In a well-known manufacturing establishment five employees were recently stricken in one day with 'Spanish influenza.' Immediately a prescription of this remedy was compounded and a bottle given to every member in the establishment, with directions to take one teaspoonful every two hours the first day, afterward three times daily. Since that date not one member of the establishment has been afflicted. And yet strenuous business has kept them employed night and day. Possibly this result is exceptional, but it is no less a fact." The formula given the employees consisted of a half-ounce of boneset, five drops of aconite, and four ounces of distilled water.

In the Lloyd Brothers' survey, 30 physicians listed boneset as the single most important remedy for the influenza, and 92 of the 222 responding identified it as one of the six most important remedies. It was considered less useful in pneumonia. One physician noted that the choice of the "most important" remedy in influenza varied from patient to patient but that boneset fit more cases than any other remedy. Another physician used boneset "from start to finish," and sometimes gave it as a tonic after the acute stage of the disease was over. In the very early stages where the patient only complained of aches and pains, this physician immediately gave large doses of boneset *often*. He was convinced that many influenza cases were aborted by the early use of boneset.

A physician who saw ten to 35 influenza patients a day during the epidemic began treatment by mixing two teaspoons of boneset and one teaspoon of pleurisy root in a cup of hot water. This was given immediately with a second dose 15 minutes later, a third half an hour later, and a fourth dose an hour after the first dose. He reported that this treatment typically reduced a fever of 103-104 degrees by three to four degrees in a few hours. Yet another physician reported that boneset was always a significant remedy in influenza.

Dosage

Eclectic dose: Five-60 drops of Specific Medicine (SM); infusion one to four fluid drams.
Moore: 20-40 drops of tincture in hot water, three times a day.

AHPA safety rating: Class 4, insufficient data available.

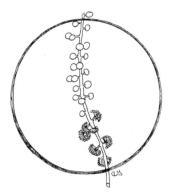

Actea racemosa
aka Cimicifuga racemosa, macrotys
(Black cohosh)

Historically, black cohosh root was primarily used as an analgesic. Native American tribes used it to relieve arthritic pain but also used it as a tonic and a remedy for colds, cough, and consumption.

Today, black cohosh is famous for easing negative symptoms of the peri-menopausal experience. Naturopathic physicians, however, are still taught that it can be one of the better remedies for ovarian pain as well as for muscle and intercostal pain.[63] Herbalists also use black cohosh as an analgesic to relieve rheumatic and neuralgic pain.[64] One clinical study shows that black cohosh, combined with other herbs, may provide some pain relief in arthritis.[65] The root contains salicylic acids.[66]

Eclectic View Of Black Cohosh

One of the first Eclectic uses for black cohosh, learned from the Native Americans, was for putrid sore throats. It came into general use by the Eclectics around 1850. "Few of our remedies have acquired as great a reputation in the treatment of rheumatism and neuralgia."[67] They used it for any dull, tensive, intermittent pain, soreness in muscular tissue and especially for pain over the abdomen. Where there was pain with fever and inflammation, it was combined with aconite or veratrum, and sometimes pleurisy root. Where the serous tissue was inflamed, it was combined with bryonia. If the pain was burning, it was combined with rhus. Black cohosh was described as "promptly curative" for the headache of influenza. In tuberculosis, it was used to lessen cough, soothe the pain (especially aching under the scapulae), lessen secretions, and lessen nervous irritability. It was used to relieve a variety of fevers. Dr. Harvey Felter called it the most important remedy to relieve muscular discomfort, and when combined with boneset —both in liberal doses—was the best remedy for the intense muscular aching and "bone-breaking" pains at the onset of influenza.[68]

Use In Pandemic Influenza

In the Lloyd Brothers' survey, nine physicians listed black cohosh as the single most important remedy they used in the 1918 pandemic. Over half of the physicians (114) listed it as one of the six most important herbs used.

In cases of flu, there is nearly always acute inflammation of the pharynx. This inflammation often causes considerable pain that is aggravated by talking or swallowing. Black cohosh in one-half to one drop doses and bryonia in relatively large doses every hour or two was used to relieve that pain.[69] One physician noted that he treated 200 cases of influenza, without complications using gelsemium, black cohosh and eyebright. He estimated that 75% of all influenza cases could be handled with these three herbs alone. After bringing down the fever with gelsemium, he would switch to ten to drops *each* of gelsemium and black cohosh in four ounces of water, administering one teaspoon every two to three hours.[70] Dr. William A. Mundy recommended black cohosh for all cases in which the patient stressed the symptom of muscular soreness; he also used it in the early stages of pneumonia to alleviate the aching.[71]

Dosage

Eclectic: The Eclectics used rather small doses of black cohosh, often one-tenth of a drop to 20 drops SM. They usually mixed ten to 30 drops in four ounces of water, dispensing one teaspoon every two hours. However, they also noted that fuller doses, short of producing headache, are very effective and the amount given to an adult could be increased to a dram or fluid ounce.

Moore: Ten to 25 drop doses of tincture, three times a day.

AHPA safety rating: 2b, not for use in pregnancy, 2c, not for use while nursing.

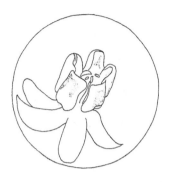

Asclepias tuberosa L.
(Pleurisy root, butterfly weed)

The root of this plant has a very long history of use for respiratory problems – hence its common name, "pleurisy root." It is also called "butterfly weed" because of the Monarch butterfly's fondness for it.

Native American tribes used pleurisy root for pleurisy, pneumonia, influenza, and other respiratory ailments. Contemporary herbalists and naturopathic physicians use it to treat respiratory infections, reduce inflammation, and promote expectoration.[72] Pleurisy root is often used today for influenza where there is a tight feeling in the chest or a painful cough. Herbalist Michael Moore notes that pleurisy root is useful in pleurisy and mild pulmonary edema because it increases fluid circulation, lymphatic drainage, and cilia function.[73]

Pleurisy root is diaphoretic which makes it useful in fevers.[74] Its diuretic and diaphoretic effect may be due to constituents that strengthen the heart contraction and allow fluid removal as a result of improved circulatory force.[75]

There is no clinical research on pleurisy root. It should be used cautiously in individuals taking cardiac glycoside drugs (such as digoxin) because it may possibly increase the risk of drug toxicity. However, some herbalists believe that it is such a feeble cardiac stimulant that it should not have a synergistic effect on heart and blood pressure medications but caution against combining it with anticholinergic drugs (such as ipratropium (Atrovent®) and oxitropium (Oxivent®).[76] It is contraindicated in pregnancy, and may cause vomiting but this occurs only at rather high doses.

Eclectic View Of The Plant

The Eclectics considered pleurisy root to be a very safe remedy because, even if used without the proper indications, it did not cause harm. At worst, it simply did not produce the desired result. Pleurisy root was widely used because it acts as a diaphoretic, diuretic, laxative, tonic, carminative, expectorant, and probably has antispasmodic action as well.

Pleurisy root works well as a diaphoretic, no matter how high the fever, because it is not a stimulant. It normalizes secretion through the skin, and may be used even if the patient is perspiring heavily. It was considered an excellent remedy for ordinary colds, and was one of the Eclectic's best remedies for catarrhal conditions caused by recent colds. In catarrhal troubles, they used dilute doses. They even used pleurisy root in sniffles, or acute colds, in infants. It was considered as good as *Euphrasia officianalis* (eyebright) or *Matricaria recuita* (chamomile) for infants. In treating tuberculosis, they used it to alleviate coughing and irritability of the mucus surfaces.

Although pleurisy root works to reduce high fevers, the Eclectics thought it was best for moderate fevers where the skin is moist and where the pulse is vibratile but not too rapid.

If the pulse is very rapid and weak, they often combined it with small doses of aconite. If the pulse was rapidly bounding and strong, they combined it with veratrum.

According to the Eclectics, pleurisy root acts on the mucus membranes of the pulmonary tract, and makes expectoration easy. In pleuritis, they used another herb, aconite, in the early stage, followed by alternating doses of pleurisy root and bryonia. With a properly chosen sedative, it was one of their preferred remedies in the early stages of pneumonia and pleuro-pneumonia. They cautioned that pleurisy root was more an assistant to other herbs than a stand alone remedy in pneumonia. Where there was a dry and constricted cough, they used small doses of pleurisy root with one or two drop doses of lobelia.

Use In Pandemic Influenza

In the Lloyd Brothers' survey three of the 222 physicians identified pleurisy root as the most important remedy for the 1918 pandemic. Seventy-two (1/3) listed it as one of the six most important herbs used, 89 used it as part of their pneumonia treatment.

Physicians made the following comments on its usefulness in pandemic influenza: For pectoral pains, bryonia or pleurisy root seem to work best. Pleurisy root controls inflammatory conditions within the lungs and is particularly valuable in allaying cough.[77] One physician who treated influenza for 22 years and who "failed only six times in a thousand cases" stated that pleurisy root can be used in "all pleuritic complaints."[78] Another Eclectic physician noted that, while gelsemium was the mainstay, he minimized bronchial complications by giving pleurisy root in small doses at the onset of symptoms.[79] In an article on treating influenza in the Eclectic Medical Journal, the author commented that pleurisy root was one of his favorites and he used it in all catarrhal affections, especially in children. He used it when the patient's skin was hot and dry and especially where there were pneumonia symptoms.

In a monograph, another physician reported that veratrum combined with pleurisy root will abort pneumonia in two to four days but the combination was most effective if given in the early stages.[80]

Dosage

Eclectic: One to 60 drops of SM typically administered by mixing 20 drops to one dram in four ounces of water, giving one teaspoon every one or two hours.

Moore: 30-90 drops of tincture, three times a day or two to four ounces of a cold infusion of the dried root, three times a day.

AHPA safety rating: 2b, not for use in pregnancy; 2d, may cause nausea and vomiting.

The Chief Sedatives

Gelsemium, aconite, and veratrum, were referred to as the Chief Sedatives (arterial sedatives), and they were vital in the Eclectic treatment of influenza. One physician expressly questioned whether pneumonia would develop from influenza if these Chief Sedatives were used properly. The Eclectics taught that the so-called sedative action of these remedies was in reality a gentle stimulation of the nerves controlling the heart and circulation and depended entirely on how they were used: In the smallest medicinal doses they are arterial or special sedatives; in large doses they are dangerous cardiac and circulatory depressants.

Each of these three remedies has its own special arena, and they do not exactly duplicate each other's effects. Aconite and veratrum may seem to act similarly but there are many properties peculiar to each. Thus, a dangerously large dose of aconite would be needed to do what veratrum accomplishes in small and safe doses. Full doses of aconite will bring down the full, strong pulse in sthenic disorders but only at a dose size that imperils the patient. On the other hand, if aconite is only used in low doses for patients with a small frequent pulse without capillary resistance, according to the Eclectics, it is a very safe remedy that may be used with great confidence.

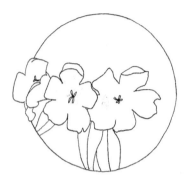

Gelsemium sempervirens (L.) J. St.-Hil.
(Yellow jasmine, yellow jessamine).
PROFESSIONAL USE ONLY

Gelsemium continues to be used by professional herbalists and naturopathic physicians to treat fevers associated with influenza, muscular weakness, myalgia, flowing pulse, apathy, deliriousness and/or hysteria.[81] Michael Moore teaches that it cools the brain and decreases wasteful fever in adults. It is helpful for the person with red eyes, flushed face, overly acute hearing, skin hypersensitivity, and agitation with lots of blood to the surface.[82] French herbalists use gelsemium for neuralgic headaches but they caution that its use requires a delicate hand because of its potential toxicity. They recommend a dose of 15 drops three or four times a day.[83] German phytotherapists find it useful as a cardiac sedative for extrasystoles and functional heart disease.[84]

Modern research supports that gelsemium has valuable, potent effects on the nervous system. Low doses of gelsemium root extracts have been demonstrated to protect mice against neurological damage and gastric erosions induced by stress.

A fluid extract of gelsemium root has also demonstrated anti-seizure ability in rats with epilepsy induced by lithium and pilocarpine injections

Eclectic View Of Gelsemium

Through the woof and warp of the Eclectic use of gelsemium runs the thread of administering it for nervous excitation and unrest, often with fever, spasm, and pain. In proper doses it was used to relax extreme nervousness and muscular tension. By diminishing the velocity of blood delivery to the head and spinal tract, it prevented spasms. It was used for hyperemia and was avoided in congested conditions.

It was considered the specific remedy for the highly feverish state with nervous excitation, for the child with a hot head and tremulous, jerky muscles, for great restlessness with elevated temperature, for the touchy, grouchy, and feverish individual who magnified his ailments, and for those who dreaded even the simple tasks of life. It was considered a powerful anti-spasmodic, second only to lobelia and potassium bromide, and it was sometimes combined with both of them.

The Eclectics said the specific indications for gelsemium's use were highly accurate: The flushed face, bright eye, contracted pupil, increased heat of the head, great restlessness and excitation. It was not considered hyperemic but was said to be indispensable in some kinds of inflammation and fevers. It was considered highly useful in the early stages of acute meningeal inflammations but was not continued beyond the sthenic stage.

In the right symptom picture, gelsemium was reported to be one of the best remedies for the spasms of childhood or infantile convulsions. It was a remedy for pain if the patient displayed nervous tension. Gelsemium was one of their favorite remedies for myalgia due to muscular exertion or due to recent colds from exposure to inclement weather. It was not given to patients with dull eyes, dilated pupils, and an expressionless face.

Many Eclectics advised that a tincture made from the fresh root of gelsemium was vastly superior to that made from the dried plant. John Uri Lloyd wrote: "For thirty years or more, Eclectic physicians have insisted that the green drug [fresh herb] possesses qualities entirely absent in the dry. This we accept without reserve, and for decades have worked only the green drug, believing that the point as concerns its superiority is not debatable...."[85]

Use In Pandemic Influenza

Gelsemium was far and away the remedy most often named as useful in the 1918 pandemic. In the Lloyd Brothers' survey, 68 physicians listed it as the single most important remedy. Eighty-seven percent (193/222) included gelsemium as one of the six most helpful remedies. It was also highly praised for its benefit in pandemics before the one in 1918.

"Fever should be controlled by the special sedatives with veratrum and gelsemium often more useful than aconite."[86] "If the patient displays marked restlessness, flushed face, bright eyes, and evidences excited cerebral excitation, gelsemium should be added or used instead of aconite or veratrum."[87]

"With boneset and gelsemium almost the whole range of

symptoms of influenza may safely be brought under control. Only when there is a known damaged heart need one be specially careful in the use of gelsemium....Study these two drugs faithfully before an invasion comes and by thus being prepared, you will be doubly armed to battle the foe."[88]

Gelsemium became the standard influenza treatment based on its stellar performance in the French Hospital study. (See chapter Did Eclectic Remedies Work?) One physician with many years of experience treating influenza favored gelsemium in patients with a high fever, intense head ache and body aches along with extreme restlessness and sleeplessness. [89]

Safety Considerations

According to the Eclectics, the smallest active doses (five to 15 minims of the specific medicine or fluid extract) cause a languid sense of ease and slight lowering of the force and frequency of the pulse. Larger doses cause a desire to lie down and cause vertigo, disturbed sight, and sometimes orbital pain. Continued small doses may, after several hours, cause vomiting but otherwise it has little or no effect on the stomach or bowels.

The cardinal symptoms of poisoning are ptosis, diplopia, dropping of the lower jaw, and absolute muscular prostration. Death takes place from centric respiratory paralysis and almost simultaneous arrest of the heart. In poisoning, the emetic or stomach pump should be used if the patient is not too weak. Tannic acid (or strong infusion of tea) should be administered, external heat applied, and artificial respiration should be used as soon as breathing shows signs of failure. Atropine can be used to stimulate the respiratory function, and ammonia, ether, alcohol and digitalis (the first three in the order named) can be used to sustain the heart until the digitalis, which should be given at once, has time to act. The Eclectics noted that morphine may antidote gelsemium but reported that this assertion had not been adequately tested as gelsemium poisoning was quite rare despite its extensive use.

Dosage

Eclectic: SM: one-tenth to ten drops of SM, usually administered by mixing ten drops to one dram in four ounces of water, one teaspoon every one to three hours.

French Hospital Study: Nine drops of gelsemium tincture, five drops of belladonna tincture, and ten grains of potassium citrate mixed in one dram of orange syrup and one ounce of Aqua Chloroformi, one dram given every four hours for the first 24 hours, thereafter one-half dram every four hours until the patient's temperature returned to normal.

Moore: Two to ten drops of tincture.

AHPA safety rating: Not covered.

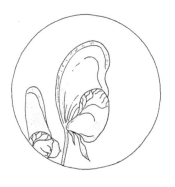

Aconitum napellus
(Aconite)
PROFESSIONAL USE ONLY

Aconite has a long history of use as a poison. Medea poisoned Thesus with aconite after he deserted her. Alexander the Great was to be lured into kissing a woman who had coated her lips with a lethal dose of aconite after acclimating to the poison by taking small doses of the plant over a long period of time. However, the assassination plot was foiled by Aristotle. Pope Adrian VI was murdered with it and the prophet Mohammed may have narrowly escaped death by aconite when he gave away a piece of poisoned meat. The deaths of Claudius and his son Britannicus are both attributed to aconite. Native American tribes also recount using aconite species as a poison and for witchcraft.[90]

Several Native American tribes identified the root as a poison but also used the root in fevers and other acute conditions. Information on how Native Americans prepared and dosed the plant was not located.

Aconite is not widely used presently but continues to be used for pain relief in neuralgia, particularly trigeminal neuralgia. Dr. Rudolf Weiss taught that it was the first remedy that should be tried in trigeminal neuralgia.[91] Michael Moore taught that aconite can be applied cautiously as a topical in trigeminal neuralgia. Moore also used aconite topically and internally, combined with *Leonuris cardiaca* (motherwort) or *Scutellaria* spp. (skullcap), for shingles, herpes zoster pain, and the "horrible skin pain" of adult chicken pox.[92] Moore taught that aconite is a hot, dry, peripatetic skin sensorium medicine. Too much of it will decrease respiration, and aconite *should not* be used on a constant basis. He used it more for sharp, neurogenic pain than for fever.

Dr. William A. Mitchell Jr., ND, combined one part aconite, three parts goldenseal, and four parts mullein and puts four drops of the mixture in the ear up to four times daily to relieve earaches. It "consistently relieves earache in about 15 seconds." In cases of neuralgia, he recommended aconite tincture at a dose level of one drop three times daily.[93]

Virtually all of the scientific research on aconite is on the toxicity of isolated constituents. Thre are a number of studies on the processed form of aconite used in Traditional Chinese Medicine, which is a very different medicine. A number of aconite's many alkaloids have shown analgesic effects in animal studies.[94]

Aconitine, a toxic alkaloid, is found in the roots of aconite. Other toxic alkaloids are found in the above ground parts of the plant. Aconitine is a potent and quick-acting poison that slows heart rate and lowers blood pressure. Aconite can be absorbed through the skin with possible fatal consequences.

Aconite and aconitine have toxic effects on the visual system in the rabbit model, including myelo-optic neuropathy. This condition can be countered by intravenous high-dose methylprednisolone.[95] Aconite contains a number of flavonol glycosides with free radical scavenging and antioxidant activities in vitro.[96] Deaths by aconite have been described in accidents, suicides, and homicides.[97] [98]

The strength of aconite varies greatly from one growth location to another, a greater variation than that between different aconite species. Michael Moore recommended consistently harvesting the plant from the same location to ensure a known strength of the medicine.

Eclectic View of Aconite

"It is capable of great good in the hands of the cautious and careful therapeutist, and is capable of great harm if carelessly or thoughtlessly employed."

Aconite was specifically indicated for patients with a small and frequent pulse, whether corded or compressible, with either elevated or depressed temperature as long as sepsis was not present. Other specific indications for the use of aconite include the following: (1) Irritation of mucous membranes with vascular excitation and determination of blood; (2) hyperemia; (3) chilly sensations; and (4) skin hot and dry with frequent, small pulse. It was used in the early stage of fevers whether the patient was restless or not.

Aconite was widely used in febrile disorders, often in combination with other herbs. The Eclectics referred to aconite as the "pulsatilla of the febrile state" and "the child's sedative." It was considered safe if used appropriately in minute doses.

Aconite was primarily (and almost solely) used in the early and acute stages of febrile disorders. The hallmark for its use was a small, fast pulse and a hot, dry fever. A classic indication was sudden onset and rapid evolution of a febrile state where it was only used in the first few days of the invasion. It was not used in more septic or chronic conditions. It was rarely (or never) used in protracted, typhoid or enteric fevers. In exanthemata, it was use to facilitate timely eruption, lower temperature, protect secretory organs, avert spasms and damage to the kidneys and the nervous system. In asthenia, it was used to moderate the force and frequency of the heart, increasing its power while lessening pain and nervous irritation. In neuralgic conditions, it was used both topically and internally.

The Eclectics used aconite topically to reduce pain, inflammation and itching. It was used cautiously, however, because it is readily absorbed through the skin. It was primarily used in acutely inflamed, painful conditions. In the Eclectic view, aconite's pain relief was accomplished by quieting inflammation. They used a diluted spray of aconite in peritonsillar abscess (quinsy), faucitis, and tonsillitis.

Aconite was considered contraindicated for congested states. Thus, it was not used in mastitis once pus had formed, in pleurisy once effusion was present or in septic fevers or any fever involving pus. In pleurisy, it was often combined with bryonia, but only bryonia was continued once effusion occurred. It was considered to act well with ipecac or rhus in gastric irritation with diarrhea and in gastroenteritis.

Aconite's action as an analgesic was attributed to its ability to reduce inflammation. In minute doses it was considered to stimulate the vascular system to achieve normal activity and reduced febrile states by correcting or regulating innervation.

In small doses, aconite quiets hurried breathing but the Eclectics were well aware that large doses could cause death through respiratory paralysis. High temperature is lowered by aconite. The kidney function is slightly increased but the skin is markedly influenced depending on the quantity administered. The motor nervous system is not noticeably affected at therapeutic doses but the sensory nerves, especially at the periphery, are notably impressed by therapeutic doses. Aconite does not act strongly on the cerebrum. On the skin and mucous surfaces, it acts first as an irritant, and then as an anaesthetic.

The mechanism of eliminating aconite was not well understood by the Eclectics but they thought it was largely oxidized because its action was of short duration. The Eclectics believed that the systemic effects of aconite seldom last over three hours although its therapeutic effect could be permanent.

Use In Pandemic Influenza

In the Lloyd Brothers' survey, 52 physicians listed aconite as the single most important remedy. Well over half (170 of 222) physicians surveyed listed it as one of the six most important herbs. The only herb mentioned more frequently was gelsemium.

The French Hospital study concluded that aconite lacked benefit in influenza but this conclusion is suspect. The Eclectics considered aconite very useful in certain specific symptom pictures (acute fever with rapid pulse) and highly contraindicated in more congested states (such as pulmonary effusion). Both symptom pictures could occur in the same patient as the disease progressed. In the French Hospital study, aconite was given randomly, regardless of the patient's particular symptoms; it is possible that aconite's benefit at one stage of influenza was masked by the lack of benefit, or harm, in a different stage of the disease.

Aconite was reported to be of value in pandemics that preceded the 1918 pandemic.[99] In one earlier epidemic, the flu caused a marked spasm of the air passages that made breathing extremely difficult, and aconite and bryonia were used to ease these spasms.[100] The 1889-1890 pandemic spread over the world in a few months. In that pandemic, where the pulse was small, wiry, feeble, and too fast (rather than full and bounding), or if chills raced up and down the spine, small doses of aconite were successful when given hourly.[101]

In the 1918 influenza, symptoms were highly varied from patient to patient but small doses of aconite were frequently appropriate if given early but "sparingly."[102] In a review of the 1918 pandemic, it was noted that patients usually were already experiencing a chill by the time they were seen by a physician. "We will find fever in the way, so we will think of our sedative. It may be aconite or veratrum. The chill will usually get aconite in small doses, frequently repeated forty minutes to one hour apart".[103] Aconite was recommended as a prophylactic "in communities where influenza has reached an epidemic stage." Five drops of aconite was added to one-half ounce of boneset and four ounces of water. A teaspoon was taken every hour the first day, and three times daily thereafter.[104]

Dr. William Mundy, in his article on the treatment of influenza, strongly recommended aconite in small doses for febrile conditions with a rapid, small pulse. "I have no fear of this remedy, even in pneumonia. In selected cases, it is one of our best remedies for pericarditis where it quiets but does not paralyze the heart.[105] "If the pulse is small, hard, rapid, skin dry, secretions deficient, the fever is best controlled by aconite. Half a drop of tincture every half hour to a child of 12 will sometimes prove highly effective in opening the skin, dissipating the fever and promoting the process of abatement of the inflammation."[106] "With adults, as a rule, I use veratrum, with children aconite. I have the best of success."[107]

Another physician noted that there were two distinct stages in the 1918 influenza. The first, "active stage" consisted of fever, flushed face, headache, restlessness and sleeplessness, and lasted for three to four days. In the second, or subnormal stage, the temperature and pulse would fall until the temperature reached a low of 95.5 and the pulse was between 42 and 58. "In this stage, I used aconite, belladonna, echinacea and cactus especially for the subnormal temperature and always with good results."[108]

One physician commented that in the first wave of the 1918 pandemic, aconite was the most frequently indicated remedy but in the second wave, gelsemium was more useful.[109] Another reported: "The recovery of influenza and pneumonia in my practice has been 100%. Early last fall, when the disease involved much mucous tract inflammation, aconite and ipecac were the most important. Of late it seems to have changed to a blood dyscrasia, for which I find echinacea the most important."[110] "I doubt we have a true pneumonia in influenza cases. There is a diffusion of blood in the lung but no pus. This has been shown in a number of aperations [sic, operations?] in local hospitals. I use bryonia and aconite."

Safety Considerations

Aconite is toxic and can be deadly. According to Michael Moore, aconite slows respiration and may be psychically disorienting. Thus, ten drops may not kill but might be too much for some people. Ginger baths, tiger balm, and other heating balms (e.g., mustard plasters, rosemary, thyme oil baths) to speed up metabolism may help antidote. But Moore says there is no true antidote and the only remedy will be physical life support.

Eclectics taught that the one diagnostic symptom of aconite poisoning is a characteristic "aconite tingling." The action of a lethal dose of aconite is rapid, symptoms coming on within a few minutes. Death may occur in one-half to six hours, the average time being a little over three hours. Treatment: Keep the patient in a recumbent position with the feet slightly elevated. If treated early, tannic acid or strong infusion of tea should be administered. Apply external heat and artificial respiration as needed. Emetics may be inadvisable due to the pressure they may place on the heart. The chief hope lies in stimulation: Ammonia or alcohol or Hoffman's anodyne, by mouth. Atropine may stimulate respiration and caffeine may stimulate the heart. A full dose of strychnine sulfate or nitrate should be given subcutaneously to sustain heart action. Adrenalin may help prevent circulatory collapse.

Dosage

Eclectic: SM ("an exceedingly poisonous and representative preparation" in its undiluted form) one-thirtieth to one-half drop usually administered by mixing one to ten drops of aconite in four ounces of water and giving a teaspoon dose every half to two hours. Tincture of aconite (1:10) one to eight minims.

Moore: 1:10 tincture of above-ground parts macerated in pure alcohol, two to five drops to four times a day. Dilute with ten parts brandy when dispensing. The roots are highly toxic; the leaves are about one-tenth as toxic. Build doses at half to one hour intervals.

Weiss: Five to ten drops or more, several times daily, ideally with the dose increasing slowly and then decreasing again.

AHPA safety rating: 3, to be used only under the supervision of an expert qualified in the appropriate use of this substance.

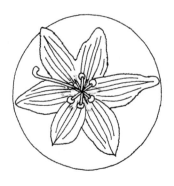

Veratrum viride Aiton
(False hellebore)
PROFESSIONAL USE ONLY

There are recent reports of veratrum poisoning caused by misidentification of the plant. In Europe, people commonly gather gentian in the spring, and the two plants look similar in the early growth stages. Patients usually experienced nausea and vomiting proceeded by a headache that began within an hour of ingestion. One of three patients developed diarrhea. Vital signs were normal except for a slow pulse (42, 45, 30 beats per minute), and electro-cardiograms revealed sinus bradycardia. Activated charcoal and antiemetics were given, and heart rates typically returned to normal within eight hours. In one patient with a heart rate of 30 beats per minute and significant hypotension, atropine and dopamine were also administered and his bradycardia and heart block persisted for about 48 hours. All patients recovered from these events.[111-113]

Naturopathic physicians use appropriate doses of veratrum at the onset of sthenic fevers if the pulse is full with marked capillary congestion. Spasms or convulsions may be present.

Michael Moore teaches that veratrum is useful for patients with fever, a strong, bounding pulse and bloodshot eyes. Often the patients cannot rest, and especially cannot lie on their stomachs without a sensation of bouncing, have red eyes, and pounding headaches. He observes that veratrum is a strong cardiac sedative, and is not a gentle herb. He considers it dangerous in more than drop doses.

Veratrum and its derivatives were used until recently to treat hypertension but was difficult to use because it has such a small therapeutic window, that is, the margin between the effective and the toxic dose was small. It was found to be useful in around 15-20% of patients with malignant hypertension.[114] Veratrum contains an alkaloid named cyclopamine. It causes a lethal fetal developmental defect, cyclopia (one eye in the middle of the face). Cyclopia occurs in sheep that eat veratrum on the 14th day of gestation. At one time in Utah, five to seven percent of newborn sheep were born with cyclopia. The formal term for cyclopia is holo-prosencephaly which means 'a single forebrain' because the forebrain and eyes of the fetus fail to separate into two symmetrical structures.

Eclectic View of Veratrum

The Eclectics viewed veratrum as a remedy of great power and value but observed that its effects were not long-lasting. Small doses yielded impressive results but had to be repeated at short intervals to maintain a continuous action. The main specific indication for veratrum is a full, bounding pulse with or without inflammation or elevation of temperature. They said it was the remedy where there is "free action of the heart" with active capillary circulation. It was used cautiously where there was gastric irritability. Fortunately, when veratrum is indicated this irritability is seldom present. Patients with acute pneumonia frequently display the specific indications for veratrum, and only bryonia was indicated more often in that ailment. In pleurisy, it was reported to sometimes act "like magic." In epidemic influenza, it was often considered the safest and most frequently indicated chief sedative.

Veratrum is specifically indicated for the following symptoms: (1) full, frequent bounding pulse, (2) full, rapid, corded or wiry pulse, (3) full, strong and intense pulse with throbbing carotids, (4) rapid pulse beating so forcefully as to interfere with sleep, (5) tissues full, not shrunken, and surface flushed with blood, (6) increased arterial tension with bloodshot eyes, (7) erysipelas resembling an ordinary infection, (8) cerebral hyperemia, (9) sthenic fevers and inflammation, (10) convulsions with great vascular excitement, full pulse, and cerebral hyperemia, (11) puerperal eclampsia, (12) red strip down center of tongue, and (13) weight in the epigastrium with forcible circulatory pulsations.

It was known as "an admirable remedy in sthenic conditions with the full bounding pulse". In all heart and circulatory disorders, especially in hypertrophy, it was used if the pulse was full, strong, and intense, the carotids beat forcibly, the eyes were bloodshot, and there was cough, headache, and weight in the upper epigastrium, while the heart might beat so violently as to shake the bed and sleep was entirely prevented.

Eclectics believed that veratrum should be studied for its ability to eliminate morbid products in many chronic ailments caused by faulty elimination. As an alterative in chronic broncho-pulmonary disorders, small doses of veratrum were sometimes given for several days and then omitted for a few days, or it was administered every other day with a syrup of lactophosphate of calcium used on alternating days. Eclectics preferred a fresh tincture of veratrum.

Use In Pandemic Influenza

In the Lloyd Brothers' survey, veratrum ranked seventh for the treatment of influenza and ranked second in number of mentions, just behind bryonia, for the treatment of pneumonia. One physician who treated at least 700 cases of influenza reported that, in nearly every case, the pulse was full and there was throbbing of the carotids. In his opinion, these symptoms called for veratrum and gelsemium, the latter in good-sized doses for its sedative effect. Another Eclectic practitioner, however, commented that he could not see why gelsemium should be combined with either aconite or veratrum. "The one indicated sedative is good practice."

Another physician reported that the first step in coping with influenza was to control fever. In sthenic cases, where the pulse is full, large and round, the face flushed and inclined to cyanosis, use veratrum. If the pulse is not over 100 beats per minute and the temperature is below 102.5, it is often possible to control the advance of the disease at once with this remedy, reducing the pulse to 60 to 65 beats per minute and hold it there until the patient recovers.[115]

Dr. Daniels wrote a monograph on veratrum. He reported that the most reliable preparations were made from the fresh root. He considered those made from dried root to be "practically useless." The dosage needed varied, and he considered that one-quarter drop up to 15 or 20 drop doses could be given with safety. "I have had patients take it in very large doses and have never seen serious results. The stomach rebels and vomiting ensues before a fatal dose is absorbed." [116]

Daniels also reported that veratrum is one of the most easily counteracted drugs and the effects of an overdose will wear off in two to three hours. He noted that veratrum is indicated when the patient is strong and the pulse bounding. However, he said he used it to good advantage where the pulse was very weak and rapid. "In slowing the heart rate, veratrum added strength to the heart beat." Combined with asclepias, it could cut short pneumonia in two to four days but the combination worked best in the early stages. He reported that nothing acts more quickly or satisfactorily in bronchitis, tonsillitis or other inflammatory conditions of the respiratory tract. It was "par excellent" when combined with gelsemium, and occasionally echinacea, for cerebral meningitis.[117]

Safety Considerations

Eclectics did not use veratrum if the patient's tongue was long, pointed, and reddened at tip, and nausea and other unpleasant gastric phenomena were present. They knew that veratrum was a powerful circulatory depressant, and that its alkaloid jervine acts directly on the heart muscle and another alkaloid, vertroidine, stimulates the inhibitory nerves and lowers the pulse rate. Jervine lowers the force of the heart and produces a more or less complete vasomotor paralysis. The emetic action of veratrum is attributed to the combined action of vertroidine and the plant resin. All vasomotor depressants, and all agents that diminish the vital force, have a synergistic effect on veratrum. Death from veratrum is caused by asphyxia.

When veratrum depresses circulation, there is marked muscular weakness and relaxation, nausea and vomiting take place and the contents of the stomach are evacuated first followed by those of the gallbladder. As a rule, purging is not produced although occasionally there is a watery diarrhea. The pulse rate has been lowered to 35 beats a minute with veratrum with a corresponding weakening of cardiac force. At this stage, emesis can seldom be prevented. In large doses it is a very dangerous agent, yet singularly, fatalities from its use were rare. In poisoning from veratrum, withdrawal of the herb and free stimulation can quickly overcome the depression. Large amounts of warm water may be given to assist emesis. This should be followed by undiluted whiskey or brandy to check the vomiting. Opium or morphine may be given by mouth or ammonia and alcoholics by enema or hyperdermic, strychnine or digitalis may be given hyperdermically. External heat, sinapism, and friction must be used and under no circumstances must the patient be allowed to rise from the recumbent position, *not even to raise the head to vomit.*

Small doses of veratrum do not appear to affect the frequency of the pulse initially but do lower its force; later, the pulse slows and becomes full and soft, and remains so unless the patient attempts to rise or make *any* exertion at which point it becomes rapid, small, thready, and sometimes almost imperceptible. Veratrum increases secretion from the lungs, kidneys, and liver but depresses the circulatory system.

Dosage

Eclectic: One-twentieth to five 1/20 – 5 drops of SM, 15 to
20 drops in four ounces of water, one teaspoon every 15, 30,
60 minutes (as required) as indicated by the pulse, and then
stopped when the pulse normalizes.

One physician reported using a slightly higher dose of
veratrum where there was a very high temperature and a full
bounding pulse: 20 drops in four ounces of water, a dram
every hour, especially in pulmonary complications.[118]

Moore: Dried root tincture (1:10, 95% alcohol), five to 15
drops up to three times a day.

Bastyr: Tincture, one to ten drops up to two times a day.
Pneumonia, one drop every 30 minutes for five to six hours to
increase emptying of the lungs.

AHPA safety rating: 3, to be used only under the supervision
of an expert qualified in the appropriate use of this substance.

NINE OTHER IMPORTANT HERBS IN INFLUENZA

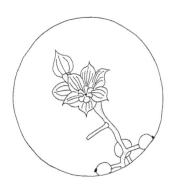

Bryonia alba L.
(Bryony, wild hops)
FOR PROFESSIONAL USE ONLY

Bryonia was called "wild nepit" in the 14th and was used to treat and prevent leprosy.

Dr. William Mitchell Jr, ND stated that he, like thousands of other practitioners, used bryonia to treat any "..itis" with characteristic pain. It is an analgesic for pains and inflammations of the serous membranes, such as those seen in the pleura, pericardium, and fascia. It is used in the later stages of inflammation where there is fever, the face is flushed and the patient is aggravated by motion or deep inhalation. It can help absorb exudates.

Michael Moore said that it is a strong herb that resolves sharp, drawing pain but that it is for extreme pain. He recommended it to help resolve inflammation and edema.

It improves healing of viscera regardless of cause. In contrast to gelsemium, veratrum, and aconite that are used for systemic heat, bryonia is for local heat.

In vitro studies show that its isolated constituents have anti-inflammatory properties.[119]

Eclectic View Of Bryonia
"An indispensable agent."

In acute diseases, the Eclectics believed that bryonia was of first importance as a remedy for pain and inflammation of the serous membranes. It is indicated for patients experiencing (1) sharp cutting or tearing pain from serous inflammation, (2) tenderness on pressure, (3) tearing pain with sore feeling in any part of the body and always aggravated by motion, (4) moderately full or hard wiry vibratile pulse, (5) headache from frontal region to occiput, (6) soreness of eyeballs on movement, (7) hyperesthesia of scalp or face, (8) hacking or racking cough, and (9) lethargy, tired, apathetic feeling, "too tired to think" and perspiring on slight movement.

In fevers, it works best where the patient is decidedly apathetic, and the tendency is toward sepsis and delirium. The patient cares little whether he recovers or dies. There is a dry tongue, sordes, a deepened hue of the tissues, capillary circulation is sluggish, and there may be a frontal headache. Chilliness is not uncommon and there is a tendency to sweat easily. In diseases of the respiratory tract and pleura, bryonia heads the list of useful remedies. It is a splendid agent for chest colds. It is the most decidedly efficient remedy in acute pleurisy where it not only subdues pain, it also lowers the temperature and overcomes capillary obstruction, thus freeing the disordered circulation. After the acute symptoms subside, it can be continued to prevent or absorb effusion.

The type of cough that bryonia relieves is laryngotracheal; frequently dry, hacking, rasping or explosive. Tensive sharp pains are almost always present, and secretion, if any, is small in quantity, consisting of a white or brown frothy mucus sometimes streaked or clotted with blood.

The Eclectics would often combine bryonia, or alternate it, with aconite for patients with acute pleurisy and a small quick pulse. In acute pleurisy with a full bounding pulse, they would combine, or use it in alternation with, veratrum.

Use In Pandemic Influenza

In the Lloyd Brothers' survey, 19 physicians considered bryonia their single most important remedy, and 162 of the 222 responding identified it as one of the six most important remedies. It ranked first in the treatment for pneumonia.

In an 1892 influenza epidemic, an Australian physician described his use of bryonia in a 45 year old woman with a history of a weak heart. Her tongue was broad and slightly pale, her pulse full with wave drops. She was very despondent, her face pale, and she had a hacking, tearing cough. Her expectoration was streaked with blood. He gave her a combination of *Pulsatilla* spp. (20 minims) and bryonia (ten minims) in four ounces of water, dosed every hour with bicarbonate of soda drinks, and continued this dose for three days after which he administered tonics.[120]

One Eclectic physician noted that bryonia and pleurisy root seemed to work best for pectoral pains, and that bryonia was most frequently indicated for the soreness of the eyeballs, the distressing frontal headache, and cutaneous hyperaesthesia. He noted that both of these herbs control inflammatory conditions within the lungs and are particularly valuable in allaying cough. He considered bryonia especially useful where the cough is dry, irritating, rasping, and every effort is accompanied by pleuritic pain.[121]

Another physician recommended bryonia for contusive pains in the back and limbs and otitis media with accumulation of fluid in the tympanic cavity.[122] Commenting that influenza almost always involves inflammation of the pharyngeal tissue, another doctor recommended bryonia where there were pharyngeal manifestations with much pain that often increases when swallowing or talking.[123]

In the 1898-1890 pandemic, bryonia was recommended for headache, especially centered in the frontal region, deep in the orbits, with soreness of the eyeballs, pain and discomfort on movement, and a lethargic, tired feeling.[124] In that pandemic, it was reported to be the most generally indicated cough remedy (used instead of "nauseous mixtures and syrups") and was reported to be the best remedy to ward off threatened pleurisy, pneumonia, and bronchitis – as well as relieve them when established. Its specific indication was sharp pain. [125]

A physician who had treated "influenza for 22 years" believed bryonia was the second great remedy after gelsemium. "The sooner you begin its use in a given case, the sooner you will cure your patients." He used it in patients with symptoms of acute catarrh, an almost unendurable headache and joint aches, a constant, harassing, uncontrollable cough, and pains about the chest symptomatic of pneumonia and pleurisy. He continued, "influenza patients will be cured if pneumonia and pulmonary complications are prevented. Bryonia and lobelia can be used as a prophylactic to prevent pulmonary complications. "[126] The first indication for bryonia was sharp, quick, piercing pain especially if increased by motion. Any hacking cough would also be improved by bryonia.[127]

Safety Considerations

The Eclectics taught that the fresh root is a strong irritant and, if bruised, may blister the skin but it was still used as a fresh plant tincture. In overdose events it causes severe gastroenteritis and has caused death. Symptoms of overdose are uncontrollable diarrhea and vomiting, dizziness, lowered temperature, dilated pupils, cold perspiration, thread-like pulse, colic and collapse. Less than fatal overdoses sometimes cause bronchial irritation with cough, hepatic tenderness, increased urination with vesicular tenesmus, cerebral fullness and congestion, jaundice and depressed action of the heart. Small medicinal doses do not cause these effects. Tannin is believed to antidote any untoward effects of bryonia.

Dosage

Eclectic: One-twentieth to five drops of SM, usually administered as five to ten drops in four ounces of water, one teaspoon dose every one to three hours. One physician mentioned a dose for children of three to four drops in water.[128]
Moore: Fresh root (1:2 in pure alcohol), dried root (1:5, 50% alcohol) tinctures, both dosed at two to ten drops to three times a day; small, frequent doses preferred

AHPA Safety rating: Not covered.

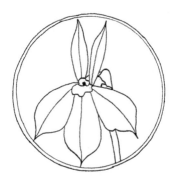

Lobelia spp.
(Lobelia)

Many species of lobelia are used as medicine. The Native Americans used *Lobelia cardinalis, L. inflata, L. kalmii, L. siphilitica,* and *L. spicata.* The Eclectics used the leaves, tops and seeds of *Lobelia inflata.* Michael Moore considers *Lobelia inflata* to be "heads and shoulders" above other species, but also uses *L. cardinalis, L. siphilitica, and L. laxiflora.* He prefers using the foliage of *L inflata* as he finds the seeds a bit too emetic. When using *L. cardinalis,* he gathers roots in the fall.

Historically, lobelia gained much notoriety through Samuel Thompson (1769-1843). Thompson used steam, emetic doses of lobelia, and cayenne (*Capsicum frutescens*) to restore body heat. He developed a series of treatments (Courses of Medicine), and the most drastic treatment was his favorite: The patient took a strong dose of an herbal tea and stood in a hot steam bath until the veins on feet, hands, and head became full. A lukewarm shower, a rubdown, and rest in a warm bed followed. The next phase consisted of a hot tea of cayenne, lobelia, and other herbs depending on the ailment and a rectal injection of the tea the patient was drinking. The tea usually caused violent emesis (if not, additional doses were administered). Refreshing herbal teas were provided in between vomiting episodes. This phase might last up to six hours and was followed by another steam, shower and cold rub down, and ended with a glass of digestive bitters. It is reported that Thompson's treatment met with great success in what was probably an epidemic of yellow fever, at least compared with the Regulars' treatments of bleeding and mercury.

Thompson was subsequently accused of sweating several patients to death but was not convicted of the charges. He went on to sell his system of medicine, and at one point claimed over 3 million followers.[129] Thompson was not an Eclectic physician.

Michael Moore taught that fresh plant tincture of lobelia is a good tonic for adrenergic stress, and that it can be used as a low level tonic for type-A personalities with poor mucus production. He said it is a good herb for those who are excitable, such as highstrung office managers. He used it in red-faced hypertensives who experience a roaring in ears when they change position, are salt reactive, and have nosebleeds in response to emotional changes. Lobelia is also good in what Moore termed "false kidney excess" - people who may be hot, red and flushed but who tend to have low blood pressure and do not accommodate blood very well (they get hot or cold easily). Lobelia can also be used to relieve stress in cases where there is self destructive, unresolved anger, grief and frustration turned inward.

Moore described lobelia as "an antispasmodic second to none." The leaves and flowers can be smoked for their antispasmodic effect on the bronchi, and can be very helpful in asthma at first signs of spasm. He comments on the safety of Lobelia: "Just stay below the nausea level and you have nothing to worry about. Where an emetic is needed, ipecac is far safer. Lobelia in excess as an emetic is dangerous."

David Hoffmann teaches that lobelia's primary specific use is for bronchial asthma and bronchitis.

A crude methanol extract of *Lobelia inflata* leaves had an antidepressant effect in mice. This action was largely attributed to beta-amyrin palmitate.[130, 131, 132] Lobeline, one of lobelia's many alkaloids, is a respiratory stimulant that activates carotid and aortic body chemoreceptors at therapeutic doses. Larger doses may produce a cough. It relaxes the tissues and favors expectoration when a large quantity of mucus is secreted. Lobeline has been used in modern medicine to treat victims of electrocution or asphyxiation, and where drug poisoning by alcohol, morphine or narcosis paralyzed the respiratory centers. It has also been used to treat asphyxia in newborns. However, due to its unpredictable effects, its use has become obsolete.[133]

Lobeline was an ingredient in a variety of drugs to aid in smoking cessation (Nicoban, Bantron, CigArest). In 1993, the FDA removed these products from the market as ineffective, and studies indicate that lobeline is not very available orally. Other studies suggest that lobeline may have potential in the treatment of methamphetamine abuse. Lobeline improves memory in rats, and improves the performance of rats in sustained attention tasks. It has been studied for its ability to function as an anxiolytic without impairing cognition or acting as a depressant.

Eclectic View Of Lobelia

The strongest indication for lobelia was a full, oppressed, sluggish, doughy pulse, especially when associated with precordial oppression, thoracic pain, soreness of chest, nausea with heavy coating of tongue at the base and fullness of tissue. Specific indications were fullness of tissue, full veins and arterial flow, lull labored and doughy pulse, sense of suffocation, dyspnea with precordial oppression, heavy, sore or oppressive pain in the chest, mucus accumulations in the bronchi, dry croupy cough. The powerfully relaxant effect of lobelia gained it a reputation as an efficient anti-spamodic. It was considered "a most admirable respiratory stimulant" when the mucus membranes were dry, or when relaxed and secretion was free but difficult of expectoration.

Lobelia was considered one of the most valuable medicines in all stages of epidemic influenza, as a vital stimulant, to regulate an imperfect circulation and to control cough and expectoration. It was considered an admirable drug in post-influenzal catarrhs if the specific indications were met.

Some conditions considered appropriate for lobelia were: (1) Pulmonary apoplexy, (2) epidemic influenza, (3) spasmodic asthma, (4) bronchospasms, (5) colds with a dry, irritative cough, (6) a non-productive, dry barking hacking cough with loud mucus rales, (7) croup, (8) pneumonia, (9) broncho-pneumonia with congestion and depressed breathing, and (10) whooping cough.

The Eclectics knew lobelia to be a powerful gastrointestinal irritant, producing emesis or, if vomiting fails, sometimes a purgative. In large doses, a state of near-collapse is induced. Small doses slow the heart but this is followed by a more or less accelerated pulse. During the depressive state, blood pressure is lowered but subsequently rises. Small doses stimulate and large doses paralyze the respiratory centers, the vagal terminals and ganglia in the bronchi and lungs. Death in animals given lobelia is due to asphyxia. However, its emetic action is usually so strong that lobelia does not act as a lethal agent. Given *in extremis*, death would more likely be due to exhaustion from vomiting than to any poisonous effect of lobelia. The emetic action of lobelia is extremely depressing and usually causes sweating. The depression, however, is of short duration and followed immediately by a sense of satisfaction and repose. The mental powers are unusually acute and the muscles are powerfully relaxed. The circulation is strengthened by small doses and enfeebled by large doses.

Use In Pandemic Influenza

Eight Eclectic physicians considered lobelia the number one remedy in the 1918 pandemic, and 79 of the 222 physicians surveyed considered it one of the six most important remedies. An overwhelming percentage of the physicians used chest applications as part of their treatment, and many of their chest applications included lobelia. (See Chapter on Chest Applications). Over half of the physicians in the survey listed lobelia as a remedy for pneumonia.

One physician commented: "Lobelia is unequalled in overcoming the oppressed condition of the chest, especially when bronchitis or broncho-pneumonia complicates the case or in croupish conditions of adults or children, or in asthmatic conditions during an attack of influenza. Aromatic spirits of ammonia with lobelia will clear up an attack of asthma.

Bryonia and lobelia can be used as a prophylactic to prevent pulmonary complication. Lobelia should be used for its antispasmodic, relaxant and expectorant effects."[134]

Dosage

Eclectic: One-tenth to drops of SM, usually administered by mixing five to 30 drops in four ounces of water, one teaspoon every one to three hours.

Moore: Lobelia inflata, fresh tincture: Five to 20 drops up to four times a day. *Lobelia cardinalis,* fresh tincture: Ten to 40 drops up to five times a day.

AHPA safety rating: 2b, not for use in pregnancy; 2d may cause nausea and vomiting, not to be taken in large doses.

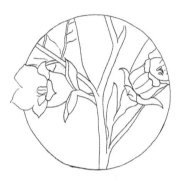

Atropa belladonna
(Belladonna)
PROFESSIONAL USE ONLY

The name belladonna ("beautiful woman") describes belladonna's ability to dilate the pupils, a human signal of attraction. Spanish women were known to use belladonna drops to enhance their allure.

The German physician Rudolf Weiss valued belladonna as the gastrointestinal antispasmodic outranking all others. He explained that, because it suppresses secretion, it is of particular value for hyperacidity symptoms. It is effective in all stomach, intestinal, and bile duct spasms. If belladonna is indicated, long-term administration is required, often for several weeks or more. Weiss concluded by saying that belladonna as an antispasmodic for the gastrointestinal tract was definitely superior to all synthetic drugs. He also commented that: "belladonna does everything the constituent atropine does so there is no advantage to the isolated constituent. It is necessary to know what one is doing when prescribing belladonna tincture. Using it correctly requires a certain amount of practice and experience."

Dr. Bastyr predominantly used belladonna as a homeopathic remedy but taught that patients with fever, a bright red face, cool extremities, dilated pupils, and excess cerebral congestion respond well to belladonna.

In a review of the medical records of 49 children with acute belladonna poisoning, the most common symptoms were meaningless speech, tachycardia, mydriasis, and flushing. In severely intoxicated children, meaningless speech, lethargy, and coma were more common, but tachycardia was less common. This review found that, although the initial signs and symptoms of acute belladonna intoxication might be severe in some children, permanent effects or deaths did not occur.[135] In 19 recumbent, healthy individuals, the administration of two hundredths (0.02) of a gram increased the frequency of breathing and swallowing-related tachycardia. In some, inspiratory tachycardia during deep, slow breathing also increased.[136] In another study, eight healthy young men took a single oral dose of belladonna tincture on four separate days. This study showed that low doses of belladonna stimulate parasympathetic activity in man, and causes vagal activation changes. The tincture had little effect on blood pressure.[137]

Low doses of belladonna had a significant protective effect on behavioral and gastric alterations induced by experimental stress in mice (e.g., locomotor, postural and exploratory activities, severity of gastric erosions, etc.).[138] In mice, orally administered belladonna had neither a sedative nor an anxiolytic effect, and did not appear to affect the central nervous system.[139]

Eclectic View Of Belladonna

The specific indications for belladonna were many: (1) dull, expressionless face with dilated or immobile pupils, dullness of intellect, drowsiness with inability to sleep well whether there was pain or not, (2) impaired capillary circulation either in skin or mucus membranes, (3) dusky, deep-red or bluish face and extremities the color being effaced by drawing a finger over the skin, the blood slowly returning in the whitish streak so produced, (4) circulation sluggish with soft, oppressed and compressible pulse, (5) cold extremities, (6) breathing slow, labored and imperfect, (7) hebetude (lethargy or mental dullness), (8) the patient sleeps with eyes partially open, (9) coma, (10) urinary incontinence, (11) free and large passages of limpid urine, (12) fullness and deep aching in loins or back, and (13) spasm of the involuntary muscles.

The Eclectics wrote: "When one observes the power of belladonna to arouse the patient from a stupid or drowsy state, or even from unconsciousness, or sees it quiet delirium, bring out the eruption, and incite the kidneys to natural action, the power of small doses of powerful medicines becomes convincing even to the most skeptical. The action of belladonna in scarlet fever is one of the strong arguments in favor of specific as compared to gross medication."[140] In neuralgia with circulatory excitement and elevated temperature, as well as in severe cases of sore throat (red, raw, swollen, intensely sore, difficulty swallowing, dryness) belladonna was often combined with aconite .

Use In Pandemic Influenza

In the Lloyd Brothers' survey, five physicians listed belladonna as the single most important remedy, and 48 of the 233 physicians considered it one of the six most important remedies. It was, however, not often discussed in articles published on pandemic influenza. One physician recommended using belladonna if there was initial primary congestion or where the pulmonary engorgement was unusually severe. "This remedy is indicated where the skin is cool, where the extremities are cold, with high temperature, where the pupils are dull and the patient is inclined to listlessness or stupor it is a very important remedy. It acts very well with veratrum and can act well with aconite although the characteristics for belladonna do not often coincide with an aconite pulse."[141] Another commented that in the second stage of influenza there was a drop in body temperature and pulse rate. This physician used aconite, belladonna, echincacea, and especially cactus "for the subnormal temperature and always with good results."[142]

One physician used belladonna to relieve the congestion found in 60% of his cases. Another, who treated influenza daily from October 1918 to January 1919, commented that "A few cases need belladonna." Yet another who treated 400 cases without a death commented that "belladonna is a wonderful drug to the physician who has mastered drug action."

In the French Hospital study, many patients benefited from the administration of belladonna. It was not as consistently beneficial as was gelsemium, but helped often enough that it was added to the gelsemium formula which the physicians decided to administer to all of their influenza patients. As mentioned earlier, the Eclectics considered gelsemium and belladonna to be quite opposed and to cancel each other out when combined.[143]

Safety Considerations

The Eclectics did not use belladonna in chicken pox, in puerperal convulsions, and in spasmodic coughs without congestion and capillary impairment. They used it cautiously as a topical because it was absorbed through the skin, and preferred other remedies to quell excessive perspiration.

Dosage

Eclectic: One twentieth to one drop of SM, usually administered by mixing five to ten drops of Belladonna in four ounces of water, one teaspoon every one to three hours. *Weiss:* Eight drops of tincture in water, three times a day.

AHPA safety rating: 3, to be used only under the supervision of an expert qualified in the appropriate use of this substance.

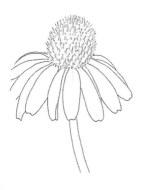

Echinacea spp.
(Echinacea)

Echinacea is a well known remedy with many different actions on the immune system. Three varieties of echinacea are used, *E. angustifolia, E. pallida,* and *E. purpurea.* The roots of *E. angustifolia* and *E. pallida* are used while the above-ground parts of *E. purpurea* are considered best for medicine. Many American practitioners believe that there are subtle but important differences in their actions, and the different varieties are often combined to capture the benefits observed in traditional use which favored *E. angustifolia* as well as the benefits of *E. purpurea* acknowledged in numerous research studies.

Echinacea was the most frequently used plant by early Native Americans.[144] It has been the subject of over 300 scientific studies.[145] Both pharmacological and clinical studies confirm that remedies containing echinacea can improve weakened immune defenses.[146] Most practitioners think that full doses of echinacea need to be administered frequently for optimum effect. As mentioned earlier (See chapter on Cytokine

Storms), echinacea down-regulates the abnormal cytokine production induced by viruses. Additional information on echinacea can be obtained from virtually any text on herbal medicine.

Eclectic View Of Echinacea

The Eclectics used the root of *Echinacea angustifolia*, and considered it to have "extraordinary powers." It was used to treat boils, abscesses, or glandular inflammations whether due to snake or insect venom, or from microorganisms that cause malignant diphtheria, cerebrospinal meningitis or septicemia, so called "bad blood" and especially a tendency to malignancy in acute or subacute conditions were deemed special indicators for echinacea.

In cerebrospinal meningitis, it was used for patients with a slow, feeble pulse (or at least a pulse not especially fast), a barely elevated temperature, and cold hands and feet. Headache with a peculiar flushing of the face was often present and associated with symptoms of dizziness and profound prostration. Echinacea was favored in tonsillitis and catarrhal affections of the nose, nasopharynx and other parts of the respiratory tract. It was considered unique in its ability to overcome the stench of pulmonary gangrene. If given early, it could avert a gangrenous termination in pulmonary affections.

It was a prominent remedy in fevers. The Eclectics found that it occasionally improved influenza cases, and in all patients with great frailness, it helped secure a good convalescence.

Use In Pandemic Influenza

In the Lloyd Brothers' survey, five physicians listed echinacea as the most important remedy they used to treat the pandemic, and 29 of the 222 physicians listed it as one of the six most important plants. Twelve mentioned its use in pneumonia.

Only a few of the influenza articles discuss the use of echinacea. One physician gave each of his more than 250 cases two to 20 drops (depending on age) of echinacea every two hours and then added other remedies as indicated. Another noted that "rusty sputum" appeared unexpectedly in many, many cases. He relied on echinacea to fortify the lung tissue against undue degeneration and was very satisfied with the results.[147] In 1929, a physician published an article on the use of echinacea in influenza. He reported his practice of giving echinacea from the very first day and continuing with good size doses until the temperature returned to normal and, where there was purulent expectoration, any cough cleared up. He considered echinacea to improve the body's ability to eliminate waste products and toxins, to stimulate and increase leucocytes, and to prevent secondary infections. He learned to incorporate echinacea into all cough mixtures until the cough was cured. "Give your other remedies as indicated" he noted, "but give your echinacea from beginning to end."[148]

A few years later, another author commented that echinacea should be given from the first day in influenza to build up leucocytosis, purify the patient's blood and meet any secondary invasion with a system of defense.[149]

One physician in the Lloyd Brothers' survey used echinacea in several pregnant women who delivered while afflicted with influenza-induced pneumonia: "I had several cases where women were delivered during the pneumonia of influenza. All were heavily dosed with Echinacea. One woman was delivered with a temperature of 104.5, pulse 130. Consolidation of left lung almost complete – recovery."

Dosage

Eclectic: One to 60 drops of SM, smaller doses preferred if frequently repeated. They sometimes dispensed it in water or syrup: One ounce echinacea in four ounces water mixed, one teaspoon every half hour in acute cases. If there were gastrointestinal problems glycerin was substituted for the water.

Moore: 30-100 drops of tincture, as needed.

AHPA safety rating: 1, can safely be consumed when used appropriately.

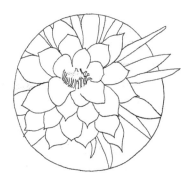

Selenicereus grandiflorus
(Cactus)

Previously this herb was known as *Cactus grandiflorus* or *Cereus grandiflorus*. Its common names include "night-blooming cactus," "night-blooming cereus," "large-flowering cactus," "sweet-scented cactus," and "queen-of-the-night." Although the Eclectics cautioned against the use of other species, modern practitioners often use *Hylocereus undatus* or *Pinocereus* spp. interchangeably. Most Western herbalists use the stems and flowers in fresh form. The Eclectics noted that the flowers were not stronger or preferable to a medicine made from stems only.

Cactus was one of Dr. John Bastyr's favorite remedies, and he used it frequently in practice. Cactus is indicated if the patient feels constriction in the chest as if iron bands were around it. (Of course, where these symptoms arise for the first time, or come on suddenly, suspect a medical emergency and handle accordingly.)

Michael Moore recommended cactus for a flighty, light-headed person with a fast, thread pulse, sense of arrhythmia, and a lost connection to the body along with fear centered in the chest, lungs, and heart. He commented that in excess, cactus may be too slowing: "All you can do is watch cartoons." It has almost no physiologic effect in small doses. Using cactus as a long-term tonic, however, is difficult today because most cardiac symptoms will be treated with prescription medicines, and possible drug interactions are unknown. Moore also reminded that, if there is constant tachycardia, there may be thyroid stress and *Lycopus Virginicus* (bugleweed) and/or *Leonuris cardiaca* (motherwort) may make the heart less responsive to that stress.

In vitro studies indicate a positive inotropic effect on isolated frog heart and the papillary muscle, probably from guinea pigs.[150] Cactine (better known as hordenine) injected intravenously in horses (200 milligrams per animal) caused an insignificant increase in heart rate for 90 seconds, oral administration (500 milligrams per animal) reportedly had no effect on circulation.[151] Experiments in intact rats, mice, and dogs show that hordenine has a positive inotropic effect upon the heart, increases systolic and diastolic blood pressure, peripheral blood flow volume, inhibits gut movements but has no effect upon the "psychomotorical" behaviour of mice. All effects are short and appear only when high doses are used.[152] One study shows that glycosidic derivatives of hordinine administered orally had a hypertensive activity in rats.[153]

Eclectic View Of Cactus
"Cactus is the only remedy that will quicken a slow heart."
"Primarily a nerve remedy, secondarily a heart remedy."

Eclectics list *Selenicereus* as "cactus" in their texts. Specific indications for its use are: (1) Impaired heart actions, whether feeble, irregular or tumultuous, (2) cardiac disorders with mental depression, precordial oppression, and apprehension of danger and death, (3) nervous disorders with feeble heart action, (4) tobacco-heart, (5) hysteria with enfeebled circulation, (6) vertex headaches, and (7) vaso-motor spasms. Two symptom pictures from their texts clarify when the Eclectics used cactus:

The patient has marked mental depression, often amounting to hypochondria and fear of impending death along with precordial weight, oppression, and difficult breathing.

The patient complains of a cord or band or a grip around the chest, around the heart or around the body. When pain accompanies this symptom, it is a lightning-like or sharp, acute or shooting pain, accompanied with a sensation of suffocation, difficult breathing, faintness, cold, perspiration or fear of impending danger.

The Eclectics used cactus for cardiac weakness due to long illness (typhoid fever, etc.), as a sedative, and for nervous exhaustion. Where there was hemoptysis with circulatory excitement, they combined it with *Lycopus* spp. They taught that cactus impresses the sympathetic nervous system and is especially active in its power over the cardiac plexus. In sufficiently large doses, it is an intense irritant to the cardiac ganglia, causing irritability, hyperesthesia, arrhythmia, spasm and neuralgia of the heart, and even carditis and pericarditis.

As with digitalis, an overdose can induce heart failure. Large doses produce gastric irritation, confusion, hallucination and slight delirium. Excessive doses cause a quickened pulse, constrictive headache or constrictive sensation in the chest, cardiac pain with palpitation, vertigo, dimness of sight, oversensitivity to noise and a disposition to sadness or paranoia. Melancholia often follows such action. Dr. Finley Ellingwood, a well respected Eclectic teacher and physician, disagreed somewhat with these teachings: "[T]here seems to be a prevailing opinion that it can be given in overdoses. I have never seen any unpleasant effects from overdoses, and I am growing into the belief that we will yet learn that there are cases where we now obtain indifferent results, or where the agent is not now advised, in which good results will be secured by much larger dosage than is now given."[154]

Use In Pandemic Influenza

In the Lloyd Brothers' survey, 64 physicians listed cactus as one of the six most important remedies. Twelve listed it as an important remedy in pneumonia.

This was a remedy primarily used more toward the recuperative phase. An Australian physician describes its use in an 1892 influenza epidemic for an elderly woman with a history of weak heart, fever, and a troublesome cough. He brought down her fever with veratrum and used lobelia to ease her breathing. Three days later, she was strong enough to sit up, was breathing with greater ease, and her temperature was down to 101 degrees but she felt nervous. He then combined veratrum (ten minim) and cactus (40 minim) for six days at which time he switched to a tonic.[155] Another physician recommended it as an herb to help reconstruct the influenza patient. He commented that physicians should not rush to digitalis when the heart is weak in action and the pulse irregular. Instead they might try *Craetagus* spp. (hawthorn), *Apocynum cannabium* (dogbane) or cactus.[156]

One physician used cactus more frequently in pneumonia, commenting: "I did not lose a pneumonia case. Seemingly they cannot die if you put on the Emetic Powder jacket heavy enough, and kept it renewed and support them with cactus".[157] Another commented: "[D]uring this pandemic, my principal remedies were gelsemium, black cohosh, and cactus to keep the heart in tone as most patients complained of weakness or dyspnea, with an occasional other remedy, as indicated. I had ten cases of pneumonia but did not lose a case.[158] Another concurred: "For weak heart action, I use cactus and nux vomica. This complication is common here."[159]

Dosage

Eclectic: One to ten drops of SM.
Bastyr: Ten to 20 drops of tincture, two times a day.
Moore: Five to 15 drops of fresh tincture, four times a day but he adds that even one to three drops can work; Ten to 25 drops of fresh *Pinocereus greggii* tincture, four times a day.

AHPA safety rating: 1, can be safely consumed when used appropriately.

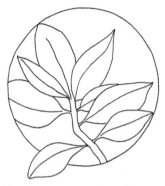

Cephaelis ipecacuanha (Brot.) Tussac
(Ipecac)
PROFESSIONAL USE ONLY

Ipecac is seldom used today by contemporary botanical practitioners although a few use it occasionally as an expectorant for bronchitis. It has largely been replaced by gentler herbs. David Hoffmann summarizes its properties and actions as follows: "In the same way that it promotes expectoration through stimulation and subsequent elimination of mucus, it fosters production of saliva. Ipecac is an expectorant, emetic, sialagogue and antiprotozoal. Ipecac remains in use as an emetic in certain cases of poisoning."[160]

Ipecac causes a release of 5-hydroxytryptamine, and is therefore used to induce nausea and vomiting. It is currently used as a model of emesis to test the antiemetic activity of 5-HT3 antagonist drugs.[161] [162] Most research on the plant concerns its use in poisoning cases.

Eclectic View Of Ipecac

Ipecac is listed as Ipecacuanha in Eclectic texts. The chief specific indications for its use are: (1) a full, broad tongue, heavily coated, with constant nausea or vomiting, and (2) irritation of the digestive tract with long, pointed, reddened tongue and tendency to nausea, vomiting, diarrhea or dysentery. They considered it useful in irritative cough and hoarseness with scanty expectoration, and in active hemorrhage. Ipecac was frequently used in patients with symptoms of irritation, capillary engorgement, and hypersecretion.

Eclectics recounted that ipecac was used in medicine in five ways: (1) As an emetic, (2) as a nauseant expectorant, (3) to check active hemorrhage, (4) to check vomiting, and (5) to control irritation and inflammation of the mucus passages of alimentation and respiration. The Eclectics primarily used ipecac to control irritation and inflammation of the mucus passages.

The Eclectics found that ipecac worked best as an anti-emetic in patients with a red, pointed tongue and evidence of irritation. However, they found it also worked where nausea was caused by foul accumulations in the stomach and the patient had a broad, flabby, slimy tongue. In the latter case, full emetic doses were sometimes given, followed by minute doses if nausea and vomiting continued.

In all abdominal conditions where ipecac was appropriate, there was a characteristic tongue (long with reddened tip and edges and prominent papillae), tenderness on pressure and the patient was noticeably irritable and easily disturbed by noises. Vascular irritability and marked hyperesthesia were also present, and the patient's senses were overly reactive and the patient was extremely sensitive to their environment.

Ipecac worked well as a hemostatic, if the blood loss was small. The Eclectics reported excellent results with ipecac in hemoptysis and hemorrhage from gastric ulcers. In those cases it was never given in emetic doses.

Allopathic physicians tended to use ipecac as an expectorant, while the Eclectics usually did not. However, when the patient had a short, irritative cough with lack of secretion or excessive secretion, they found low doses of ipecac could be useful.

Ipecac in larger doses irritates the skin and mucosa. When inhaled, it causes heat and violent sneezing. In some patients, it causes attacks that resemble asthma with great dyspnea, wheezing respiration, cough, marked anxiety and prostration often accompanied by violent and prolonged sneezing and spitting of blood with free expectoration of mucus following. In doses of less than one grain, it is a gastric tonic and hepatic stimulant. Doses of three to ten grains will cause nausea, some depression of the pulse, languor, diaphoresis, and increased mucus secretion. In doses greater than fifteen grains it is emetic. If emesis fails, catharsis may result or it may produce both emesis and purgation. Ipecac feces are peculiar – bilious and mush-like. Emetine, a constituent in ipecac, has caused death by gastrointestinal inflammation and cardiac paralysis.

The Eclectics disliked the use of ipecac as an emetic for emergency poisoning unless other emetics were unavailable. To them, ipecac's greatest value was in its beneficial effect on irritation of the gastric and intestinal mucosa when used in minute doses.

Use In Pandemic Influenza

None of the physicians in the Lloyd Brothers' survey listed ipecac as the most important remedy but 57 considered it one of the six most useful remedies. In pneumonia, it was listed by 86 physicians as a useful herb.

It was used in minute doses to quell nausea where there was no diarrhea.[163] Ipecac was sometimes combined with opium in Dover's powder, a medicine used by the allopathic physicians but not by the Eclectics who considered opium contraindicated in influenza. One physician commented: "I do not use opium in any form, believing it has killed more people in America than the German war."[164] Dover's powder was found ineffective in the French hospital study. In the 1918 pandemic, Eclectics primarily used ipecac to relieve the tendency of hemorrhage from the mucus membranes of the nose, throat or lungs that so frequently occurred.

Dosage

Eclectic: one-thirtieth to 20 drops of SM.

AHPA safety rating: 1b, not for use in pregnancy; 2d, may cause nausea and vomiting, not for long-term use, and contraindicated in cardiac disease.

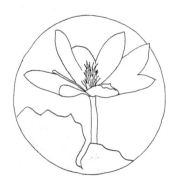

Sanguinaria canadensis
(Bloodroot)
PROFESSIONAL USE ONLY

Queen bumblebees are the primary pollinators of many early spring wildflowers, including sanguinaria. Flies, too, play an important role in transferring pollen from one flower to the next.

Sanguinaria remains in use as an ingredient in many herbal expectorant cough medicines, and its main use by herbalists today is in bronchitis. It is considered to have expectorant, antispasmodic, emetic, cathartic, nervine, and cardioactive actions. It is also widely used in mouthwashes and toothpastes, such as Viadent®, because of its antibacterial, antifungal, and anti-inflammatory activities that reduce gingival inflammation and plaque formation.[165] Its main alkaloid is antimicrobial, anti-oxidant, and anti-inflammatory.[166]

Eclectic View Of Sanguinaria

Sanguinaria is specifically indicated for burning and itching mucous membranes, especially of fauces, pharynx, eustachian tubes and ears, less frequently of larynx, trachea, and bronchi, occasionally of stomach and rectum, and rarely of vagina and urethra. It is also appropriate if the mucus membrane is red and irritable, or in patients who are nervous and have a red nose with acrid, burning discharge, constriction in fauces or pharynx, an irritative cough and difficult respiration.

It is specifically indicated in respiratory disorders when chilliness is a dominant feature as well as when there is burning and itching of the naso-laryngeal tract, tickling or burning in the nasal passages with super-abundant secretion, irritation and tickling provoking cough. When secretions are checked, it relieves dry cough by promoting normal moisture. Some allopathic physicians used it in whooping cough and croup but the Eclectics did not because the doses needed were too harsh for young children. They did use it in syrup, with or without *Lycopus, Prunus* or *Eucalyptus,* after pneumonia had been cured but the patient remained weak and had a cough and viscid secretion that was difficult to expectorate. They also used it in headache, catarrhal jaundice, and duodenal catarrh where there was feeble circulation and cold extremities.

The Eclectics also taught that the alterative properties of sanguinaria should not be overlooked, and considered it an important remedy in respiratory disorders. They reported that it resembled lobelia somewhat in action, and was a useful stimulating expectorant but only after active inflammation had been subdued. They did not use it as an emetic.

Use In Pandemic Influenza

Thirty four of the physicians surveyed considered sanguinaria one of the six most important herbs in influenza treatment, none listed it as the single most important remedy. In pneumonia, 27 listed as an important herb. In the 1918 pandemic, many patients experienced a "harassing" cough after a bout of influenza, one that could lead to broncho-pneumonia. Sanguinaria was used to soothe that cough. Sanguinaria was also an ingredient in the chest rubs many physicians used to prevent pulmonary complications from arising from influenza. (See chapter on Chest Applications.)

Dosage

Eclectic: One to ten drops of SM, usually administered as five to ten drops in four ounces of water, one teaspoon every two to three hours.
Moore: Ten to 15 drops of tincture (1:5, 60%).

AHPA safety rating: 2b, not for use in pregnancy; 2d may cause nausea and vomiting, powerful emesis is produced by as little as one gram. Contains the toxic alkaloid sanguinarine which suggests the plant should not be used in large amounts.

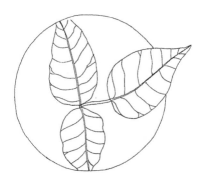

Rhus toxicodencron
(Poison ivy)
PROFESSIONAL USE ONLY

The concept of using rhus, poison ivy, as a medicine is startling to the modern mind. Rhus is not used by most practitioners, and its medicinal uses are not covered in most texts on botanical medicine. However, it remains available commercially to licensed practitioners. Interestingly, Native American tribes used rhus both topically and internally. The root or plant poultice was used topically by "skilled medicine men" on infectious or chronic sores and to cause swellings to open. Internally, decoctions were taken as an emetic, and as a tonic rejuvenator.[167]

Urushiol is the compound that triggers the well-known poison ivy rash. It binds skin protein, acting as a hapten. T-cells take up the antigen-hapten complex and present them to Langerhan's cells. These migrate to local lymph nodes where type 1 T-helper cells are activated. This activates other immune cells and leads to inflammation.

It is reported that Native Americans ate very small amounts of the new rhus leaf in the spring as a method of oral tolerization. This has been confirmed clinically.[168] Systemic contact dermatitis can occur in sensitized individuals when they are exposed orally, transcutaneously, intravenously or by inhalation. One patient developed a diffuse skin eruption after applying a homeopathic mother tincture of rhus topically while taking a homeopathic rhus preparation internally. She reacted again to the topical application in a challenge two months later while eight healthy controls failed to react to the topical application of the tincture. The mother tincture was a maceration of fresh plant in 65% ethyl alcohol. It appears that the internal homeopathic preparation may have helped diffuse the skin eruption beyond the sites of the tincture application.[169]

In Korea, rhus sap or lacquer (from *R. verniciflua, R. trichocarpa* and *R. javanica*) is ingested to treat gastrointestinal problems and as a health food, usually in cooked chicken. Many cases of systemic contact dermatitis have been reported from such ingestion. [170]

Urushiol (in an urushiol-ethanol microemulsion) selectively and profoundly inhibited the growth of ovarian cancer cells and only negligibly affected normal cells at the same concentration.[171] An ethanol extract of rhus significantly inhibited 5-lipoxygenase in vitro.[172]

Eclectic View Of Rhus

Rhus was used for nervous irritation, nervous tension, and the typhoid state. Its chief indication was a long-pointed tongue with prominent papillae, associated with burning heat, redness, and great unrest. Other indications include:

(1) A patient with a moderately quick, small, sharp pulse with great restlessness with or without vomiting, (2) a child that starts from sleep with a shrill, frightened cry, tongue red and irritable, and the presence of red spots, (3) strawberry tongue, (4) burning pain, (5) acrid discharges from the bladder or bowels, (6) brown sordes, (7) red, glistening erysipelas with burning pain, (8) conjunctival inflammation with pain, photophobia and burning lacrimation (tears) and (9) old ulcers with shining red edges.

The Eclectics taught that the great unrest that requires rhus is similar to that which gelsemium relieves, but the gelsemium patient is hot, agitated, has great mental excitement, bright eyes, and contracted pupils. With rhus, the nervousness takes on the form of twitching, jerking and seems more motor than mental alone. The sharp, shrill cry of the rhus patient 'once heard, will never be forgotten.' This brain cry was said to be frequently heard in grave disorders such as typhoid fever and meningitis. The secretions of the rhus patient are lacking, unless there is diarrhea. Frontal pain, sharp in character, is another prominent indication for rhus, and great unrest with vomiting is one of the most direct indications for its use especially when there is a rhus tongue: Reddened on tip and edges, perhaps of a strawberry character, and sordes on the lips and teeth. Rhus is also of value in gushing diarrhea. Rhus was used to relieve pain of a burning character, whether deep or superficial.

The tincture of rhus was treated with lead salts to remove the uruschiol and prevent rashes when the tincture was prescribed. Large doses of rhus cause stupefaction or a sort of intoxication with vertigo, impairment of the special senses, papillary dilation, chilliness, sickness at the stomach with thirst and burning pain. In rhus overdose, the pulse becomes slow, irregular and small, sometimes convulsions ensue. A pint of rhus berries caused drowsiness, stupor, delirium, and convulsions in two children who ate them. The root infusion caused skin rash, a harsh cough, scanty urine, and severe gastrointestinal symptoms in another patient. Topically, rhus is a powerful irritant poison. The Eclectics taught that rhus acts strongly on the nervous system and can be an ideal sedative to control excited circulation. They considered it of great value in children's diseases.

Use In Pandemic Influenza

In the Lloyd Brothers' survey, rhus was not listed as the single most important remedy but was listed by 25 physicians as one of the six most important herbs. Nine listed it as an important remedy in the treatment of pneumonia.

One physician advised the use of rhus, added to a sedative mixture, if the patient starts or jumps at the least noise, has a unilateral headache, and the tongue is long, pointed, and with prominent papillae.[173] Another reported using rhus for a strawberry tongue, frontal headaches and for the excited nervous condition of a child.[174] Dr. John Scudder commented that rhus was "an epidemic remedy" that was frequently used in some influenza epidemics but hardly at all in others. The indications for its use in influenza are frontal head pain, sharp stroke of the pulse, bright flush on left cheek or in spots, burning pain, especially superficial, and a peculiar redness of the papillae of the tip of the tongue.[175]

One physician commented that the Chief Sedatives (gelsemium, aconite, and veratrum) on occasion failed, even though clearly indicated, until rhus had been used first.[176]

Dosage

Eclectic: Usually administered as five to 15 drops in four ounces of water, or one teaspoon every hour in acute disorders, and four times a day in chronic. It should as a rule be given as a simple. As mentioned, the Eclectics for the most part used lead salts to remove the uruschiol from the tincture. Dr. John Scudder did not use this process for his tinctures yet did not report any adverse effects from his tinctures. He simply prepared a fresh tincture (1:2, 98% alcohol). Tinctures sold today are made with a low alcohol content to avoid extracting uruschiol.

AHPA safety rating: Not covered.

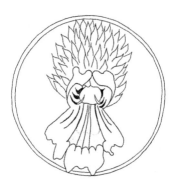

Euphrasia officinalis
(Eyebright)

Eyebright is a tiny plant that only grows in northern countries like Sweden and Finland. It is becoming rare in the wild, and other herbs should be substituted for eyebright whenever possible. It remains a popular topical treatment for relief of redness, swelling, and visual disturbances in acute and subacute inflammations such as conjunctivitis. Naturopathic physicians are taught to use it in catarrhal diseases of the upper respiratory tract, such as cold and flu. It is said to provide almost instantaneous relief for sniffles in young infants. It is widely used as a treatment for hay fever.

Eclectic View Of Eyebright

The Eclectics used eyebright for acute catarrhal ailments with copious discharge of watery mucus. They used it in influenza epidemics to control the profuse lachrimation (excess tearing of the eyes) that occurred in many epidemics. The whole plant was used as medicine.

Use In Pandemic Influenza

Eyebright was not one of the primary remedies used to treat the more serious symptoms of influenza. It was combined with aconite when the catarrhal phase of the influenza provoked extreme tearing of the eyes.[177] However, one physician relied heavily on eyebright. He reported successfully treating 200 cases of influenza with a combination of gelsemium, black cohosh, and eyebright, and he felt that probably 75% of all influenza cases could be treated with these three herbs. In cases with a cough, runny eyes, sneezing and a watery discharge, he gave ten to 60 drops of eyebright in four ounces of water, one teaspoon every three hours.[178] Another physician used it for symptom relief, especially in children.[179] Yet another used a dose of eight drops every hour and found it to give prompt but temporary relief of nasal symptoms.[180]

Dosage

Eclectic: One to 60 drops of SM.
Moore: 30 to 90 drops of dried plant tincture (1:5, 50%).

AHPA safety rating: 1, can safely be consumed when used appropriately.

Honorable Mentions

Twenty other herbs for influenza

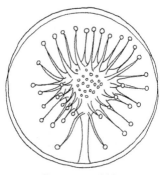

Drosera rotundifolia

Influenza presented itself in many different ways. It varied from pandemic to pandemic, and it varied with time during each pandemic. It expressed itself differently in different patients. Different physicians had different approaches to the disease and there were some in the survey whose practice included both Eclectic and Regular approaches. As a result, many remedies came into play during treatment. Those mentioned more than once in the Lloyd Brothers' survey, or mentioned as helpful in Eclectic textbooks, are discussed briefly in this chapter.

Baptisia tinctoria
(wild indigo)

Small clinical trials show that baptisia, combined with herbs such as echinacea, safely and effectively reduced the duration of upper respiratory infections in a clinical study of adults.[181] In patients with severe bacterial bronchial infections, antibiotics administered with an herbal formula that contained baptisia and echinacea led to a faster recovery than the use of antibiotics alone.[182] The Eclectics considered baptisia specifically indicated for (1) patients with fullness of tissue, leaden, purplish or livid discoloration, tendency to ulceration and decay (gangrene), (2) sepsis with enfeebled circulation, (3) fetid discharges with atony, (4) with a swollen, bluish face that looked like it had been frozen or long exposed to cold, and (5) typhoid conditions. Baptisia was, as a rule, not used in acute diseases showing great activity but was considered distinctly useful in septic conditions. An important indication was disintegration of tissue. Six of the physicians in the Lloyd Brothers' survey considered baptisia an important remedy, one considered it important in the treatment of pneumonia.

Dosage

Eclectic: One to 20 drops SM, usually administered as 20 drops in four ounces of water, one teaspoon every one to two hours.

Moore: Ten to 25 drops of fresh (1:2, 98%) or dried (1:5, 65%) tincture to three times a day.

AHPA safety rating: 2b, not for use in pregnancy; 2d, not for long-term use except under the supervision of a qualified practitioner.

Cinnamomum spp.
(cinnamon)

Cinnamon is a common spice that has been approved to treat loss of appetite and dyspepsia by a German regulatory agency (the German Commission E). Cinnamon is also commonly used as a hemostatic agent. The Eclectics used it specifically for passive hemorrhages. They also valued its antimicrobial properties in colds as well as epidemic influenza. They considered it a very important remedy for hemoptysis of limited severity. It was often combined with *Lycopus virginicus* to control passive bleeding from the lungs.
Two of the physicians in the Lloyd survey used cinnamon oil rather than cinnamon tincture.

Dosage
Eclectic dose: Five to 60 drops of SM; one to five drops of cinnamon oil.
Moore: 20 to 40 drops of dried plant tincture (1:5, 60% alcohol, 5% glycerin), four times a day.
AHPA safety rating: 2b, not for use in pregnancy.

Collinsonia canadensis
(stone root)

Collinsonia remains in use primarily as a treatment for hemorrhoids and other disorders resulting from pelvic congestion. The Eclectics used the fresh root and plant. Primary indications for its use were irritation with a sense of constriction in the larynx, pharynx or anus. They felt it worked best where there was a feeble or sluggish venous and capillary flow. It was considered a highly effective medicine for laryngitis brought on by overuse of the voice but they also considered it valuable in other forms of laryngitis. Four of the surveyed physicians considered collinsonia one of the most important remedies in the 1918 influenza pandemic.

Dosage

Eclectic: One-tenth to 30 drops of SM or tincture
Moore: 20 to 40 drops of fresh tincture (1:2, 98%), to three times a day or 45 to 60 drops of dried plant tincture (1:5, 60%) to four times a day. The dried plant tincture is inferior.
AHPA safety rating: 1, can safely be consumed when used appropriately.

Corallorhiza spp.
(coral root)

The Eclectics described corallorhiza as the most perfect diaphoretic, even surpassing pleurisy root in action. It was favored over *Jaborandi* spp. because it did not depress the heart. It was viewed as particularly valuable in the declining stages of bronchopneumonia for prostration after coughing spells, with copious, heavy expectoration, and great weakness. It was the "ideal remedy" for convalescence after influenza. It was also valuable for dry bronchial irritation with wheezing, and paroxysms of an irritable cough. Then, as now, *Corallorhiza* was scarce in the wild virtually precluding its use as a medicine. "It is to be regretted that its extreme scarcity makes corallorhiza an almost unobtainable drug."

Dosage

Eclectic: One to two drams of tincture made from four ounces of root in a pint of dilute alcohol or whiskey.

Moore: 30 to 90 drops of fresh (1:2, 98%) or dried (1:5, 60%) tincture in hot water.

AHPA safety rating: Not covered.

Digitalis lanata
(fox glove)
PROFESSIONAL USE ONLY

Digitalis is the plant that gave us the prescription heart medicine digoxin. Although practitioners are still trained in the indications for the use of digitalis plant, only a few still use it, often for patients who cannot tolerate prescription heart medicines. Eclectic physicians were well versed in its indications and contraindications, and it was their foremost heart medicine. "Digitalis cases, it must be remembered are those which are helped greatly or moderately, those in which no good effect may be expected, and those in which it is dangerous, or at least harmful." It was used to counteract heart weakness following septic fevers and pneumonia. It was not valued as a febrifuge, and was not recommended as a sedative in fevers and inflammations. It could, however, be used to strengthen a weak heart after an infection if the specific indications for its use were met.

Eclectics generally did not recommend its use in influenza: "When the heart action is weak in action and slightly irregular, do not rush to digitalis. Consider crataegus, cactus or apocynum."[183] Another Eclectic wrote: "In fever with prostration, weak pulse, weak heart, cactus is unsurpassed. When the heart is on the point of failure or in the asthenic part of the disease is the only time digitalis or strychnine should be used in doses sufficient to produce an immediate effect."[184] Five physicians listed digitalis as one of the six most important herbs they used in influenza, 13 listed it as a remedy used to treat pneumonia. The only physician who explained his use of digitalis in influenza stated: "I attribute my success to the fact that I have practically treated every case of influenza as though it were complicated with pneumonia. Sustained the heart with Veratrum, Digitalis or Nux, and kept the patients quiet."[185] Other physicians suggested that cactus was a far superior remedy than digitalis for patients weakened by influenza and would accomplish the same results in a more benign way.

Dosage

Eclectic: One-fifth to one drop of SM. One to ten drops of digitalis tincture (1:10).

AHPA safety rating: 3, to be used only under the supervision of an expert qualified in the appropriate use of this substance.

Drosera rotundifolia
(sundew)

Drosera continues to be used to treat certain coughs. Dr. Rudolf Weiss notes that it acts well and synergistically with thyme in whooping cough. However, drosera is a tiny plant that is challenged in the wild, and only cultivated drosera is appropriate for use today. If the source cannot be verified, substitute one of the many other herbal cough remedies. Eclectics used drosera for expulsive or explosive spasmodic cough with dryness of the air passages, whooping cough, and uncontrollable, irritating cough. They thought it was less useful in the coughs of bronchitis.

Three of the physicians in the Lloyd Brothers' survey listed drosera as one of the six most important influenza remedies; one thought it the most important remedy, and none mentioned its use in pneumonia. One of the physicians surveyed, however, wrote: "Am lost without Drosera in these 'flu' cases."[186] Another physician wrote that it was highly useful to control explosive, barking coughs with little secretion or fever in convalescence.[187]

Dosage

Eclectic: One-tenth to ten drops of SM.

Weiss: One to five drops of tincture in combination with other herbs. He noted that drosera's spasmolytic properties only come into play when the dose administered is small.

Moore: Five to 15 drops of fresh (1:2, 98%) tincture, to four times a day.

AHPA safety rating: Not covered.

Hydrastis canadensis

(goldenseal)

Goldenseal was used in catarrhal states of the mucus membranes where there was no acute inflammation. It was also used to stimulate gastric and intestinal secretions as it was considered one of the most effective bitter tonics. Eclectics used it to sharpen appetite and stimulate digestion rather than as an antimicrobial, its primary use today. In the epidemic, its effects on digestion were used to "reconstruct the influenza victim." Two physicians listed it as one of the six important herbs in influenza. Goldenseal is challenged in the wild, and only cultivated goldenseal should be used.

Dosage

Eclectic: One to 30 drops of SM.
Moore: 15 to 30 drops of fresh (1:2, 98%) tincture or 20 to 50 drops of dried (1:5, 70%) tincture, to four times a day.
AHPA safety rating: 2b, not for use in pregnancy.

Hyocyamus niger
(Henbane)
PROFESSIONAL USE ONLY

Hyocyamus was indicated for patients with nervous irritability, unrest and insomnia; dilated pupils and flushed face with debility, delirious fevers, spasmodic and convulsive coughing, and as a remedy to relieve pain, spasm, and nervous unrest especially in the aged, the frail and weak, and in infants. Two physicians listed it as one of the six important herbs in influenza.

Dosage

Eclectic: One-tenth to 20 drops of SM.
Moore: Three to ten drops of fresh (1:2, 98%) or dried (1:5, 50%) tincture, to three times a day.
AHPA safety rating: Not covered.

Inula helenium
(elecampane)

Inula is an aromatic root used as a stimulating expectorant and tonic. It was widely used by Native Americans for coughs, lung disorders, asthma, chest pains, fevers, and as a tonic to strengthen the digestive organs. It remains a popular herb for dry irritative coughs, to soothe irritated throats, and for lingering respiratory infections. The Eclectics favored it for bronchial irritation, with cough of a persistent, teasing character with copious expectoration.

None of the physicians in the Lloyd survey mentioned inula. However, the texts taught that inula, as a syrup, was especially useful for the cough that persisted after a bout of influenza. The syrup was made by boiling an ounce of inula root in a pint of water until eight ounces remained, then one-half pound of sugar was added. One physician reported using ten drop doses of inula every two hours "for gangrene of the lung."[188]

Dosage

Eclectic: One to 60 drops of SM. One to four drams of inula syrup.

Moore: Ten to 30 drops of fresh (1:2, 98%) or dried (1:5, 60%) tincture, to four times a day.

AHPA safety rating: 2b, not for use in pregnancy; 2c, not for use while nursing. Large doses cause vomiting, diarrhea, spasms and symptoms of paralysis.

Iris versicolor

(blue flag)

FOR PROFESSIONAL USE ONLY

The roots of this plant were used as an alterative, to promote repair and removal of waste from the body. Specific indications for its use included nausea and vomiting or regurgitation of food; enlarged lymph glands, and muscular atrophy and other wasting of the tissues.

It was listed as one of the six most important remedies by only one physician but he listed it as *the single most important remedy for influenza.*

Dosage

Eclectic: One to 20 drops of SM.

Moore: Five to 20 drops of dried plant (1:5, 80% alcohol) tincture to three times a day.

AHPA safety rating: 2b, not to be used in pregnancy; 2d, may cause nausea and vomiting.

Lycopus virginicus

(bugleweed)

Lycopus today is mainly used to treat hyperthyroidism. The Eclectics used it more broadly. The specific indication was as a sedative where the heart lacked power and the pulse was frequent. It was highly valued in the advanced stages of acute disease with great debility, and was considered a safe herb that had many of the effects of digitalis. It was deemed "preeminently useful" in passive pulmonary bleeding. The Eclectics often combined it with cinnamon and ipecac to

control such bleeding, a condition that occurred frequently in
the pandemic. The textbooks referenced this use, but it was
not mentioned in the Lloyd Brothers' survey.

Dosage

Eclectic: One to 60 drops of SM.

Moore: 15 to 40 drops of fresh (1:2, 98%) tincture, to three
times a day.

AHPA safety rating: 2b, not for use in pregnancy; 2d,
contraindicated in thyroid enlargement or hypothyroid, and in
simultaneous administration of other thyroid treatments.

Strychnos nux vomica
(nux vomica)
PROFESSIONAL USE ONLY

This medicine is made from the seeds of a tree. The seeds
contain the alkaloids brucine and strychnine. Dr. Rudolf
Weiss reports that the tincture of nux vomica still has a role
to play in herbal medicine. In small doses it is only a tonic
bitter with all the virtues of the same. Bitter tonics are used in
dyspepsia, especially after infectious illnesses, and are used to
stimulate appetite. Dr. Weiss preferred to label his tinctures
"nux vomica" on prescriptions as patients often were troubled
by the word *Strychnos*, strychnine being known as a powerful
poison. When dispensing this tincture, it should be added
to a large amount of water as the bitter taste will otherwise
be too strong.[189] Naturopathic physicians primarily use
nux vomica as a gastrointestinal stimulant but also use it in
urinary incontinence in the elderly and children as strychnine

increases sensory excitability and heightens muscular excitability. This includes excitation of the muscles involved in peristalsis. They consider it a very useful medicine when used carefully.[190]

The primary Eclectic use of nux vomica was as a restorative tonic bitter to improve digestive function and appetite. This use would have been common among allopathic physicians as well.

In the Lloyd Brothers' survey, nux vomica was listed by nine physicians as one of the six most important herbs but it was not listed by any as the single most important remedy. It was mentioned by 14 as important in the treatment of pneumonia.

In 1892, an Australian physician reported that he typically gave a tonic that included 20 drops of nux vomica as a restorative treatment after an influenza epidemic.[191] Another physician reported after the 1918 pandemic that extreme prostration was met with nux-vomica. "This remedy has been abused so much that I almost abandoned its use long ago but I learned to regard it highly during this recent experience. It certainly did great work in supporting the patient during the prostration that attended and in hastening convalescence and, I believe, guarding against relapse."[192] In an article titled "after influenza," another physician noted that, of the medicines that would help in reconstructing the flu victim, nux-vomica was the one most likely to be abused. "It and its alkaloid, strychnine, are generally used as a whip to stimulate. It should be used chiefly for the gastric affections with hepatic involvement that often follow influenza....Give it until improvement is well begun and then discontinue its use. Switch to Hydrastis if there is still gastric weakness with hydrochloric acid if an acid is needed or capsicum if there is evident lack of normal secretion."[193] In influenza, one physician recommended its use "sometimes" for subnormal temperature and rapid, weak action of the heart.[194]

Dosage

Eclectic: One-thirtieth to five drops SM, usually administered as five to 15 drops in four ounces of water, 1 teaspoon every one to three hours.

AHPA rating: Not covered.

Passiflora incarnata
(passionflower)

The leaves and stems of this beautiful flowering vine are used to make medicine. The Aztecs used the leaf to treat insomnia and anxiety, and these uses were adopted into European medicine where passionflower is a common ingredient in remedies for sleep, nervous stomach ailments, and nervousness. Eclectics liked it as a rest producing remedy especially in the very young and very old. They also used it as an antispasmodic in whooping cough and asthma. Both uses might have been of value in influenza. It was mentioned once in the Lloyd Brothers' survey and in an article suggesting its use for sleeplessness in influenza.[195]

Dosage

Eclectic: One to 120 drops of SM.
Moore: One-half to one-and-one-half teaspoons fresh (1:2, 98%) or dried (1:5, 50%) tincture, to four times a day.
AHPA rating: 1, can be safely consumed when used appropriately.

Phytolacca americana
(poke)
PROFESSIONAL USE ONLY

Phytolacca is still widely used to treat catarrh, tonsillitis, laryngitis, swollen glands, mumps, and mastitis. Eclectics considered it specifically indicated for hard painful glandular enlargements, and pallid sore throat with cough and difficult respiration. "Without phytolacca we should be at a loss to know how to treat glandular affections undergoing swelling or inflammation." It was useful in laryngitis, chronic catarrh, and other acute and chronic mucus affections. Eight physicians considered it one of the six most important herbs in influenza.

Dosage

Eclectic: One to 20 drops of SM, usually administered as ten to 30 drops in four ounces of water, one teaspoon every one to three hours. One to 30 drops of recently dried root (1:2, 76% alcohol) tincture.

Moore: Five to 15 drops of fresh tincture (1:2, 98% alcohol).

AHPA safety rating: 3, to be used only under the supervision of an expert qualified in the appropriate use of this substance.

Pilocarpus jaborandi
(jaborandi)
PROFESSIONAL USE ONLY

Jaborandi is a shrub that grows in Central and South America. It has been termed a "genuine" diaphoretic in that it directly and powerfully stimulates both the sweat glands and the salivary glands. Dr. Rudolf Weiss considered that, in ordinary cases, its action was too powerful and carried too great a risk of toxic side effects. He reserved the use of jaborandi for rare conditions that failed to respond to other treatment. The Eclectic specific indications for jaborandi were: (1) deficient secretion, (2) marked dryness and heat of the skin, (3) muscular pain and spasm, (4) suppression of urine where the urine was dark and of a high specific gravity, (5) pulse hard, full, sharp and strong with deficient secretion, (6) dry, harsh cough, and (7) belladonna poisoning. The keynote for its use was suppressed secretion of any type but the Eclectics cautioned that it had to be used very carefully. Jaborandi has a depressive action on the heart and can, through excessive diaphoresis, cause debility. In respiratory ailments, the Eclectics preferred to combine it with other indicated remedies such as bryonia, asclepias, and lobelia. In the Lloyd Brothers' survey, four physicians considered it one of the six most important influenza remedies.

Dosage
Eclectic: One to 60 drops of SM.
Moore: 15-30 drops of dried (1:5, 60%) tincture in warm water.
AHPA rating: 2b, not for use in pregnancy.

Podophyllum peltatum
(may apple)
PROFESSIONAL USE ONLY

Podophyllum was not a widely used Eclectic remedy for influenza. In fact, its use may have been primarily by physicians with a more allopathic belief in the need to purge patients to initiate recovery. In small doses, the Eclectics found it useful for atonic forms of indigestion where the patient also complained of dizziness, loss of appetite, and heavy headache. It was used to counter constipation which apparently was common in some influenza patients. Four physicians listed it as one of the six most important remedies.

Dosage

Eclectic: One-tenth to 30 drops of SM, fractional doses preferred.

Moore: Ten to 20 drops dried (1:5, 95%) tincture. He cautions against its use in overt disease or in physical depression.

AHPA *safety rating:* 2b, not for use in pregnancy.

Polygala senega
(seneca snakeroot)

This herb is indicated for relaxed respiratory mucosa and skin, with hoarse cough, excessive secretion, mucus rales, nausea and vomiting as well as for the cough of bronchitis. It has an acrid taste and leaves a disagreeable sensation when swallowed. It may be used in subacute forms of cough as is found in chronic bronchitis with profuse secretion. It was contraindicated in fever, and was little used by the Eclectics.

It was an ingredient in "the vicious preparation, Coxe's Hive Syrup" which was reformulated into syrup of squill. In the Lloyd Brothers' survey, one physician considered senega an important remedy, and one used syrup of squill.

Dosage

Eclectic: One to 20 drops of SM.

Moore: Ten to 45 drops of fresh (1:2, 98%) or dried (1:5, 65%) tincture, to four times a day. Small, frequent doses work best.

AHPA safety rating: 2b, not for use in pregnancy; 2d, contraindicated in gastritis and gastric ulcers. Not for long-term use.

Pulsatilla spp.

(pulsatilla)

PROFESSIONAL USE ONLY

Pulsatilla was used for a variety of emotional states including insomnia with nervous exhaustion, pain with debility, fear of impending death as well as for many physical issues such as deep-seated heavy pain in the globe of the eye, headaches, and orchitis. It was not usually used to treat acute inflammations but small doses were beneficial when the described emotional states appeared in a patient with acute inflammation of the nose, fauces, larynx or bronchi. In colds where the eustachian tubes were stuffed and occluded, it was alternated with gelsemium.

Three physicians listed it as one of the six most important remedies in influenza.

Dosage

Eclectic: One-tenth to ten drops of SM, usually administered as five to 30 drops in four ounces of water, one teaspoon every two to three hours.

Moore: Three to ten drops of fresh (1:2, 98%) tincture only, to four times a day.

AHPA rating: Not covered.

Sticta pulmonaria
(lungwort moss)

The Eclectic textbooks recommend sticta to relieve muscular pain accompanying catarrhal fever and epidemic influenza. The chest soreness it relieved was increased on breathing and felt like that arising from a bruise or overexertion. It was useful for the pain of coughing. Three of the physicians surveyed considered it one of the six most important herbs in the pandemic.

Dosage

Eclectic: One-tenth to ten drops of SM.

Moore: 20 to 30 drops of dried (1:5, 60%) tincture, to four times a day.

AHPA rating: Not covered.

Stillingia sylvatica
(queen's root)

Michael Moore described stillingia as an energetic expectorant and an immunostimulant above the diaphragm (lungs, face), that tends to bring on a healing crisis in slow conditions, i.e., facilitates getting sick. It is an herb for the cold and depressed, not hot, anabolic and organized. Its only specific use is in chronic sore throats. Stillingia is a subtle but strong medicine that is not for excess or acute stages except when used as a cough drop. Eclectics considered it an important alterative "when a good preparation can be procured." It was used when there were feeble tissues with slow removal of broken down material and slow reconstruction of tissue, mucosa red, glistening and tumid with scanty secretions, skin lesions with irritation and ichorous discharge, laryngeal irritation with paroxysmal hoarse croupy cough, post-faucial irritation with cough or irritative winter cough. It was considered more valuable as part of a chest application (See Chapter on Chest Applications).

Five of the physicians surveyed mentioned stillingia as an important herb, far more reported using it in chest rubs.

Dosage

Eclectic: One to 30 drops of SM.

Moore: Ten to 30 drops of fresh (1:2, 98%) or dried (1:5, 50%) tincture, preferably small frequent doses.

AHPA rating: 2c, not for use while nursing.

CHEST APPLICATIONS

The vast majority of the physicians answered the Lloyd Brothers' survey question on chest applications affirmatively, and considered them important to ward off pulmonary complications in influenza. Only six of the physicians did not, and three failed to answer the question.

Historically, chest rubs and applications were widely used by physicians and lay folk alike. There is no explanation for when, or why, this practice was discontinued but they are not commonly used today. No research indicates that they lack benefit. In fact, animal research indicates that volatile oils (often found in chest rubs) penetrate the lung tissue and have a strong antimicrobial action. A recent study showed that Vicks™ salve applied to the chest enhanced lung clearance in patients with chronic airways obstruction.[196] It would therefore seem like an appropriate way to deliver antimicrobials to the lung tissue, especially where congestion is impeding circulation and the delivery of compounds through the blood. Perhaps their lack of popularity is due to the fact that they can be messy.

The vast majority (164) physicians surveyed used a product manufactured by Lloyd Brothers, Libradol. Libradol came in different strengths. The mild Libradol was made for topical use in infants and "supersensitive persons." The regular Libradol contained a mixture of *Symplocarpus foetidus* (skunkcabbage), *Sanguinaria canadensis* (blood root), *Cephaelis ipecacuanha* (ipecac), *Melaleuca cajuputi* (cajeput), *Lobelia spp.* (lobelia),

Laurus spp. (laurel), *Capsicum annuum* (cayenne) and *Nicotiana tobacuum* (tobacco) in a "plasma" that could be easily spread on parchment or directly on the skin. Libradol did not soften or run with the heat and moisture of the body. A recipe for Libradol is not available, nor is the product. It was often used to ease pain in the chest.

Many other topical applications were mentioned, and counter-irritants such as turpentine were also commonly used. Often the choice was based on what was available in the patient's home, sometimes the choice was based on what was available to the physician. Several noted that they did not have access to Libradol during the pandemic.

Poultices (cataplasms) are preparations designed to be applied externally to relax, hold moisture, and allay pain and inflammation. They should always be removed without being permitted to dry. Chest applications were applied to the back as well as the chest, to cover both sides of the lung area, and were usually applied warm.

Emetic Powder, compound powder of Lobelia, powder of lobelia: *Lobelia* spp. powder, six drams; *Sanguinaria canadensis*, powder three drams; *Symplocarpus foetidus*, three drams; *Cephaelis ipecacuanha* powder, four drams; *Capsicum annuum* powder, one dram. Mixed.

The Eclectics describe this powder as an exceedingly efficient local application to the chest for colds and general broncho-pulmonary troubles. It was sprinkled on a larded or oiled cloth and applied warm.

This chest application was, after Libradol, the most popular chest rub. The Emetic powder was considered an invaluable application to the chest in acute thoracic diseases. It was reported to give marked relief from pleural and muscular pains and to alleviate the sense of suffocation and fullness accompanied by a feeling of soreness within the chest. Its effects when applied locally in broncho-pulmonic affections were highly valued by the Eclectics.

The Eclectics did not know how it worked, and stated that, while its action could not easily be explained, its positive effect was "a well attested clinical fact and its certainty makes it a remedy that we will not be likely to part with." It was widely used in acute bronchitis, pleurisy, pneumonia, pleurodynia, and soreness of the pectoral walls. The Eclectics taught that the emetic powder could be freely used without danger of unpleasant consequences, and was preferred over heavy poultices that could be uncomfortable for the patient. They often recommended wearing a cotton jacket (prepared by lining an undershirt with a uniform layer of cotton) over the larded cloth for best effect. Petrolatum was substituted for other greases by some physicians.

Stillingia liniment: One fluid ounce of oil of stillingia, one-half fluid ounces each of lobelia oil and cajeput oil, and two fluid ounces each of alcohol and glycerine. Mix in the order given. Stillingia liniment is prone to precipitate and often thickens to a magma or jelly. It should be well shaken before use. If it has solidified, it should be replaced with a fresh supply. This liniment has both stimulant and relaxant properties. It is used in chronic asthma, croup, epilepsy, chorea, etc. In asthma and croup, the throat, chest, and neck should be bathed with it three or four times a day. It is a good internal remedy for irritative and chronic coughs where it is given on sugar or in syrups. In chorea, epilepsy, and spasmodic diseases, the whole spinal column is bathed with it. In asthma, its action is very prompt and effectual, relieving and ultimately curing some very obstinate cases. In the majority of cases when applied, the patient experiences a peculiar taste in the mouth.

An alternate, weaker version was often used: One-half fluid ounce of oil of stillingia, one-half fluid ounce of oil of cajeput, one fluid dram of oil of lobelia, and three fluid ounces of alcohol. Mix. Dosage: One to five drops. Amina is a modification of Compound Stillingia Liniment that adds *Anemopsis californica*.

Oil of Stillingia: Percolate the powdered root with full strength alcohol and evaporate off the percolate to a creamy consistency. It has a dark red color, a slight odor, and the taste of the drug leaves an acrid sensation in the throat and fauces that is persistent in effect. This preparation is prone to gelatinize and precipitate. Often it turns to a brown mush and should then be thrown away as useless.

Oil of Lobelia: This so-called oil of lobelia is simply a syrupy extract of lobelia made with stronger alcohol preferably acidulated with acetic acid. This so-called oil is the active constituent of compound stillingia liniment. The fixed oil of lobelia may be obtained by bruising the seeds between heated rollers and pressing while hot in a strong linen cloth between iron plates. Its consistency is like that of linseed oil.

Oil of Cajeput: Distilled from the leaves of *Melaleuca leucadendron*. It is a powerful diffusive, stimulant, diaphoretic, and antispasmodic.

Flaxseed poultice: A flaxseed poultice was frequently applied in acute pulmonary disorders. Mix four and one-half ounces of powdered flaxseed (approximately) and ten ounces of boiling water, stir constantly "so as to make a cataplasm." The British pharmcopeia advises four ounces of flaxseed poultice causes the skin to be blanched, sodden, and wrinkled.

Lobelia poultice: Take equal parts by weight of lobelia powder and *Ulmus rubra* (slippery elm) bark, add a sufficient quantity of weak, warm lye to form a cataplasm. "It should frequently be renewed." Alternatively, powdered lobelia was sprinkled on a larded cloth and applied warm. Typically used in wounds, swellings, inflammations, etc.

Antiphlogistine: Used as an external counterirritant cream for temporary pain relief of stiff and sore muscles, backache, strains, arthritic and rheumatic pain, sciatica, lumbago and bursitis.[197] It remains available commercially, primarily as a veterinary medicine for horses.

Regular Strength: Each gram contains: methyl salicylate 12.5%, camphor 1%, menthol 0.75% and eucalyptus oil 0.5% w/w, and other nonmedicinal ingredients.

Extra Strength: Each gram contains: methyl salicylate 18%, camphor 1%, menthol 0.75% and eucalyptus oil 0.5% w/w. And other non-medicinal ingredients.

The Eclectics commented: Antiphlogistine is one of our best applications in local inflammation. In pneumonia it is the best we have and should never be forgotten. [198]

Counter-Irritant: One-third part oil turpentine; one-third part oil linseed (raw); one-third part olive oil. Spread on flannel and apply. This is a useful application in croup and pneumonia etc. Lobelia powder (from seed) may be added to improve its action, especially in croup and pneumonia.[199]

Onion poultice: Three large fresh, organic onions and distilled water. Slice the onions thinly and sauté them in a small amount of distilled water until transparent. Fold half into a diaper or similar piece of cloth so that the finished pack is approximately eight by eight inches. Apply to the chest as hot as can be tolerated and immediately cover with a towel to hold in the heat. Begin preparing another poultice with the other half of the onions. When the first one is cool, immediately replace it with the second. After treatment, gently dry the chest and tuck the patient into bed to rest. Roasted onion makes an efficient poultice for acute broncho-pulmonic inflammations, especially of young children, when local applications are desired. Onion poultices are objectionable only when made too heavy, carelessly applied, or when applied to open surfaces.

Onion poultice is used in cases of deep lung congestion and bronchial inflammation. It will bring penetrating relief when it hurts too much to cough. It can also be applied over the ear and lymph nodes to treat ear aches; then the poultice is made smaller in size.[200]

This was a commonly used home remedy as the ingredients are easy to obtain. It was considered to be quite effective.

Juniper Pomade (modified): Four ounces of dehydrated lard, five drams of paraffin, one dram of white wax, three drams of oil of juniper berries , four drams of finely powdered *Grindelia robusta*, or non-alcoholic extract, is the best proportion. Melt the paraffin and wax first, gradually adding the lard. Then add oil of juniper berries, mixing well with an egg-beater. Then add *Grindelia robusta*.

Useful in eczema, as a salve in nasal catarrh, etc. [201] The original juniper pomade was a mixture of lard, oil of juniper and Fowler's solution.

Many other types of chest applications were mentioned in the Lloyd Brothers' survey, including Vick's salve, mustard plasters, and any oily substance. One physician mentioned that, when he ran out of Libradol, he used moist heat, oil of mustard, and turpentine. In some cases, cotton or a jacket was used by itself, indicating that heat to the area was considered important, although three or four physicians preferred ice applications. However, another physician criticized the use of cold applications in pneumonia: "A most unreasonable fallacy . . . is the use of cold applications to the chest....Its influence upon the capillaries is to produce congestion, and if persisted in, stasis....On the other hand, heat applied and persisted in, over the entire diseased area, is a most potent and physiological antagonist. .. It stimulates the capillaries and physiologically unloads the venous capillaries to drive the accumulating tide of blood through the engorged vessels into the veins."

Non-Herbal Remedies

Although the Lloyd Brothers' survey asked for herbal remedies used most often in the 1918 pandemic, many physicians also included non-herbal remedies in their responses. The following remedies were mentioned as important by more than one responding physician.

Ammonium Chloride (Muriate of Ammonia): Depending on how it was used, muriate of ammonia was variously a refrigerant, laxative, expectorant, diaphoretic or diuretic. It was toxic in very large doses. It was sometimes used as a nasal spray (five to 125 grains in one ounce of water) in mucus diseases of the throat and nasal passages. Internally, it was considered a valuable remedy in broncho-pulmonary disorders. Two physicians surveyed considered it one of their most useful influenza remedies.

Aspirin and Sodium salicylate: Four physicians used aspirin while six used sodium salicylate. The Eclectic articles on influenza treatment strongly opposed the use of aspirin in influenza. The active extract of the *Salix alba* (white willow) bark, salicin, was isolated in 1828. It is highly acidic in a saturated solution with water, and is called salicylic acid for that reason. The same chemical was isolated from *Filipendula ulmaria* (meadowsweet) in 1839. This latter extract was somewhat effective but also caused digestive problems such as irritated stomach and diarrhea, and sometimes death in high doses. In 1853, salicylic acid was neutralized, creating acetosalicylic acid. In 1897, aspirin, acetylsalicylic acid, was first manufactured.[202] A physician, during the pandemic, praised sodium salicylate as a highly effective treatment while at the same time warning of the dangers of aspirin. When asked if this opinion makes sense, Dr. Eric Yarnell, ND responded: "Yes. Aspirin is a synthetic chemical, acetylsalicylic acid. It is definitely different than salicylate--for example, natural salicylates of all kinds have no effects on platelets, while ASA/aspirin permanently inhibits platelets from sticking to each other. Aspirin also cause gastrointestinal and other adverse effects like Reyes syndrome while salicylate does not, especially in the form of a whole plant. Pure salicylate can cause an ulcer and severe gastrointestinal pain, but only in very high doses."

Bicarbonate: One physician responding to the Lloyd Brothers' survey listed bicarbonate as his single most important remedy in the treatment of influenza. He did not specify whether he was using potassium or sodium bicarbonate.

The Eclectics taught that sodium bicarbonate was an excellent antacid and could be used cautiously in urinary disorders. Some used it as a treatment for sore throat, and tonsillitis. In inflammatory diseases, it suppressed abnormal increases of fibrin in the blood, and helped resolve the disease. Hemorrhagic fever and influenza in extreme cases cause a disorder of blood clotting, diffuse intravascular coagulation and leads to organ failure. An abnormal increase in serum fibrin is one aspect of that disorder, and bicarbonate is still administered, along with other drugs, in attempts to treat it.

Eclectic Dose: Five to 40 grains of sodium bicarbonate in a glass of carbonated water.

Potassium bicarbonate was specifically indicated by a leaden pallor of the tongue and mucus membranes and tremulous action of the voluntary muscles and in debility out of proportion to diseased conditions. Dose: Ten to 30 grains, well diluted.

Calcium sulphite: Calcium sulphite was chiefly used to stop fermentation by cider makers. The Eclectics rarely used it as medicine, except occasionally to disinfect and stimulate chronic, obstinate skin ulcers. Nonetheless, two physicians mentioned it as one of their six most important influenza remedies. Dose: Five to 60 grains.

Calomel (mild chloride of mercury): Internally, calomel acts as a purgative. In allopathic medicine, relatively large doses (one to three grains every three to four hours) were used as a sialagogue in febrile diseases, often combined with Dover's powder or some other opiate. In 1918, smaller (but to modern standards still toxic doses) continued to be used by mainstream medicine. Thus, the Department of the Navy – Bureau of Medicine and Surgery, issued the following advice on September 26, 1918: "If you become ill, go to bed and do not try to keep on with your work. In the average case, recovery is in 5-6 days. Keep the body warm, maintain fresh air but avoid chilling. At the beginning, a cathartic such as 2.5-3 grains of calomel followed by a Seidlitz powders or Epsom salts is useful. Aspirin in 5 grain doses is useful for pain but do not take large doses of aspirin, phenacetin or other medicines. Send for the doctor."

A few Eclectics used very small doses (two to three grains of the 3x trituration, three times a day) in lethargic states characterized by a long-continued tired feeling, with marked daytime drowsiness and nocturnal wakefulness. Three physicians in the Lloyd Brothers' survey characterized calomel as one of the six most important influenza remedies. However, most Eclectics strongly advised against *any* use of mercury.

Castor oil: Castor oil is expressed from the seed of *Ricinus communis*. The oil, taken internally, is a mild cathartic. It was a widely used home remedy until quite recently. "The greatest objections to this cathartic are its nauseous taste and its tendency to cause sickness and unconquerable disgust." Three of the physicians surveyed considered castor oil one of their six most important influenza remedies.

Codeine: Codeine (methylmorphine) is an opioid that is used for its analgesic, antitussive, and antidiarrheal properties. It is an alkaloid found in the opium poppy. Codeine was once extracted from opium but today is synthesized from morphine. Two physicians surveyed considered codeine one of their six most important influenza remedies.

Dover's powder (compound powder of opium and ipecac): Ten grains of Dover's powder contains one grain opium, one grain ipecac, and eight grains milk sugar or potassium sulphate. It was reported to be an excellent sedative, stimulant, anodyne, and narcotic with a better action than either of its ingredients administered separately. It was used as a pain relieving agent and to promote sleep, when opium could not be used alone. Dose: Two to ten grains, preferably in capsules. Most Eclectics disapproved of the use of opium in influenza but two of the physicians did use Dover's powder. These two respondents also reported using other remedies more commonly used by allopaths.

Phenacetin: Phenacetin was introduced in 1887. It was principally used as an analgesic (three to 500 milligrams per day). Its analgesic effects are due to its actions on the sensory tracts of the spinal cord. In addition, phenacetin has a depressant action on the heart where it acts as a negative inotrope. It is also an antipyretic, acting on the brain to decrease the temperature set point. In 1983, phenacetin was removed from the market because of its link to analgesic-induced nephropathy. Phenacetin and products containing it have been shown to be carcinogenic in animal models. In humans, case reports have implicated phenacetin-containing products in renal pelvic cancer. In one prospective series, phenacetin was associated with an increased risk of death due to urologic or renal diseases, death due to cancers, and death due to cardiovascular disease. Acetaminophen (e.g., Tylenol) a metabolite of phenacetin has similar analgesic and antipyretic effects but does not share its carcinogenic side effects.[203] One physician mentioned using phenacetin.

Podophyllin: Podophyllin is the resin from *Podophyllum peltatum*, the mayapple plant. It acts as a certain but slow cathartic in four to eight hours. It was usually combined with other herbs to prevent cramping. The Eclectics tended not to use it for its cathartic properties, but instead used it — in tiny doses — to stimulate the nervous system, and to improve digestion and blood making ability. The dose used was about 0.05 grains. It was considered contraindicated in patients with pinched features and a small, wiry pulse. Four physicians considered podophyllin one of their most important influenza remedies.

Potassium chlorate: Potassium chlorate should be kept in glass-stoppered bottles and *great caution should be observed* in handling the salt as dangerous explosions are liable to occur when it is mixed with organic matters (cork, tannic acid, sugar, etc.), or with sulphur, antimony sulphide, phosphorus, or other easily oxidizable substances, and either heated directly, or subjected to trituration or concussion. In very large doses, it is extremely poisonous, producing besides the effects of potash, violent local inflammation. It is a very important remedy, particularly where there is a tendency to septicemia. It seems to hold a position between ammonium chloride and potassium nitrate. It was used occasionally in malignant febrile diseases and cholera. It is diuretic.

The keynote for its selection is a cadaverous fetor of the secretions and breath. It has been efficiently employed in scorbutus, hepatic affections, in aphthous ulcerations of the mouth, *cancrum oris*, mercurial salivation, abscesses, boils, eruptions, ulcers, purpura hemorrhagica, etc. Associated with stillingia, it is a good agent in syphilis and syphilitic ulcerations of the mouth with cadaveric fetor. It is a useful agent in diphtheria when indicated but the kidneys should be carefully watched and, if affected, the drug should be withdrawn. When indicated by the cadaverous odor of the breath, and bluish, pallid membranes or ulcerated, foul discharging mucus surfaces, it is an excellent therapeutic agent in respiratory lesions. In pneumonia, with hot, pungent skin, putrid odor of the breath, and increased secretion, it may be given in five or ten grain doses every three hours. When large doses are administered, they should be given at mealtime and in a large quantity of broth or other liquid. Specific indications: (1) Puerperal troubles arising from decomposition of fragments of placenta, blood clots, and absorption of fetid lochia, (2) fetid breath, the fetor, as of decaying animal tissues, (3) pallid tongue, pale or bluish membranes, (4) ulcerated, foul-discharging mucus surfaces, (5) tender mouth and gums, with fetid salivation, (6) tongue coated, dirty and thick, (7) cough with purulent expectoration, and (8) hot, pungent skin, and cadaverous odor of discharge. One physician surveyed felt comfortable using this explosive remedy, and, in fact, listed it as his most important influenza remedy.

Quinine: Quinine appropriately was used "as the great remedy" for malarial and other intermittent fevers. Most Eclectics, however, considered it inappropriate and even harmful in influenza. "If you give physic, nauseants, quinine, or the fashionable antipyretics, you will have trouble."[204] In their opinion, quinine required periodicity and other indications. When used inappropriately, it adds to the nervous aggravations and naso-aural disturbances.[205] "Personally we would rather trust isolation, bed rest, warm fresh air and no medication to heavy physiological doses of synthetic antipyretics, quinine, whiskey and other agents . . .We would rather use Eupatorium, Gelsemium, Bryonia, Macrotys and

Euphrasia."[206] Quinine was one of the remedies tested in the French Hospital study but found ineffective. Nonetheless, five physicians listed it as one of the six most important remedies. It was much more widely used by allopaths in the epidemic.

Sodium sulfate: Sodium sulphate was considered a mild but efficient cooling laxative or purgative. Its usual dose was six to eight drams dissolved in eight to ten ounces of water. Non-cathartic doses of ten to 20 grains in a pint of water were also given when the patient's tissues were full, pale and sodden, the tongue pallid, full and easily pitted by the teeth. Four physicians listed it as one of their most important influenza remedies.

Sodium Sulfite: It agrees well with the stomach, has no local irritating properties and acts as a diuretic. It was used as a remedy to counter the effects of mercury. The special use of sodium sulphite in the Eclectic school was for a symptom pattern commonly found in many diseases – the broad pallid tongue, with white or dirty white coating and extremely fetid breath, although fetid breath is not always present. The Eclectics taught that when these symptoms were present, the patient's prompt response to sodium sulfite was amazing. It was particularly recommended, provided the right symptoms were present in fermentative and putrefactive conditions, typhoid and other fevers, erysipelas, smallpox, tonsillitis and other forms of sore throat, herpes, scabies, ringworm, etc. The dose of sodium sulphite is from ten to 60 grains, three times a day. Four physicians surveyed used sodium sulphite.

Spirit of nitre, Lloyd's nitre: Lloyd's nitre, freshly made, carries five percent by weight of the complex natural ether produced by the reaction between nitric acid and alcohol. This ether is only partly nitrate of ether as it contains other substances that are formed as incidental parts of the reaction. Spirit of nitrous ether was frequently employed in Bright's disease, congestion of the kidneys, and painful affections of the urinary apparatus. It was also deemed a good remedy in flatulent distension of the stomach, to allay nausea, and to quiet nervous agitation. It was said to lessen the frequency of the pulse, reduce the temperature, and promote secretion. For this, use one-half to one teaspoon added to a half glass of water, and given in teaspoon doses every hour. For fevers in children, mix four ounces of water with three ounces of sweet spirit of nitre, and give one teaspoon every hour. Three of the physicians surveyed listed spirit of nitre as an important remedy.

Appendix A

Glossary

Acute encephalitis: Encephalitis is an acute inflammation of the brain, commonly caused by a viral infection. Sometimes, encephalitis can result from a bacterial infection, such as bacterial meningitis, or it may be a complication of other infectious diseases like rabies (viral) or syphilis (bacterial).

Allopath: A physician who practices conventional medicine.

Analgesic: A compound capable of producing analgesia, ie, one that relieves pain by altering perception of painful stimuli without producing anesthesia or loss of consciousness.

Anodyne: A pain relieving agent, less potent than an anesthetic or narcotic.

Anticholinergic: Inhibiting or blocking the physiological action of acetylcholine, a neurotransmitter, at a receptor site

Antidote: A remedy or other agent used to neutralize or counteract the effects of a poison.

Antiemetic: A medicine that prevents or controls nausea and vomiting.

Antimony: Antimony is a chemical element (Sb). Clinically, antimony poisoning is very similar to arsenic poisoning. In small doses, antimony causes headache, dizziness, and depression. Larger doses cause violent and frequent vomiting, and will lead to death in few days. Very large doses will cause violent vomiting, causing the poison to be expelled from the body before any harm is done. The Eclectics did not use antimony.

Antipyretic: An agent that reduces or prevents fever (also called a febrifuge).

Antitussive: Preventing or relieving cough.

Anxiolytic: A drug that relieves anxiety.

Aphonia: Complete loss of voice

Aqua chloroformi: Add enough chloroform to distilled water in a dark bottle to maintain a slight excess of chloroform after the contents have been repeatedly and thoroughly agitated. When required for use, pour off the needed amount, add distilled water and agitate making sure an excess of chloroform is always present. This is an agreeable vehicle for other medicines and is particularly useful in non-inflammatory diarrhea, flatulent colic, gastralgia, and other forms of abdominal pain. Because of its preservative qualities it is valuable in solutions containing organic materials which otherwise might ferment. It is a pleasant vehicle for cough mixtures, and alone is useful in coughs characterized by tickling, irritation or other nervous sensations in the bronchi and throat. Whooping cough is palliated by it. It is also used as a local hemostatic where bleeding is small. Dose from one fluid dram to one fluid ounce.

Asthenia: Weakness or debility.

Auscultation: Listening to the heart and lungs using a stethoscope.

Blood dyscrasia: Any abnormal condition of the blood.

Bronchitis: Bronchitis is an inflammation of the bronchi (lung airways), resulting in persistent cough that produces consideration quantities of sputum (phlegm).

Calomel: Mild chloride of mercury.

Carminative: A substance that stops the formation of intestinal gas and helps expel gas that has already formed.

Catarrh: Inflammation of a mucous membrane, especially of the respiratory tract.

Cathartic: A powerful agent used to relieve severe constipation (also called a purgative).

Citrate of magnesia: A white, coarsely granular salt, without odor and having a mildly acidulous, refreshing taste. It was used as a mild laxative. Dose: two drams to one ounce, well diluted.

Clinical study or trial: A rigorously controlled test of a new drug or a new invasive medical device on human subjects.

Conjunctivitis: Inflammation of the eye or eyelid

Controls (in a clinical trial): A study in which the experimental procedures are compared to a standard (accepted) treatment or procedure.

Cutaneous hyperaesthesia: Hypersensitivity of skin, especially to pain.

Cyanosis: Bluish discoloration of the skin or mucous membranes caused by lack of oxygen in the blood.

Dover's powder: Opium powder ten grains, camphor powder 40 grains, ipecac powder 20 grains, potassium bitartrate 160 grains, mixed. The

Eclectics said this was an excellent anodyne and diaphoretic, perhaps superior to any other preparation in its diaphoretic effects. It favors perspiration without augmenting the heat of the body. Dose: Three to five grains every three to five hours in febrile or inflammatory diseases, and in some cases ten grains three times a day. Its action may be materially promoted as a diaphoretic by warm drinks, such as catnip, balm or sage tea, lemonade etc. but not immediately after administering the powder so as not to provoke vomiting. Some practitioners substituted *lactucarium* or twice the quantity of *cypripedium* resin in place of opium. Potassium nitrate or sodium bicarbonate is sometimes substituted for the potassium bitartrate.

Diaphoretic Powders: Substitute for Dover's powders. Diaphoretic powders are made by combining powdered pleurisy root, ipecac and camphor. The Eclectics considered this powder safer than Dover's powders, but said it retained all the anodyne and sedative effects of the latter.[207]

Diaphoretic: An agent, taken internally to promote sweating (also called sudorific).

Diplopia: Double vision.

Dram: A unit of apothecary weight equal to an eighth of an ounce. It is also equal to 60 grains

Dyspnea: Shortness of breath, difficult or labored breathing.

Edema: Excessive accumulation of fluid.

Emesis: The act of vomiting.

Emetic: A medicine that induces nausea and vomiting

Epistaxis: Nose bleeds.

Erisypelas: A bacterial skin infection usually affecting the arms, legs, or face, characterized by shiny, red areas, small blisters, and swollen lymph nodes.

Exanthemata: A skin eruption or breaking out, as in measles, smallpox, scarlatina, and the like diseases -- sometimes limited to eruptions attended with fever.

Expectorant: A substance that stimulates removal of mucous from the lungs. Stimulating expectorants "irritate" the bronchioles causing expulsion of material. Relaxing expectorants soothe bronchial spasm and loosen mucous secretions, helping in dry, irritating coughs.

Faucitis: Inflammation of the fauces which is the passage from the back of the mouth to the pharynx, bounded by the soft palate, the base of the tongue, and the palatine arches.

Febrifuge: An agent that reduces fever (also called an antipyretic).

French Hospital Study Formula: This formula combined nine minims (drops) of gelsemium, five minims of belladonna, ten grains of potassium citrate, one dram of orange syrup and one ounce of aqua chloroformi. One dram (about one-eighth of an ounce) was given every four hours for the first 24 hours, and one-half dram every four hours thereafter until the patient's temperature returned to normal, at which point the formula was discontinued. The potassium citrate was added as a mild diuretic.

Glyconda: The Eclectics used Neutralizing Cordial, a combination of goldenseal, turkey rhubarb, cinnamon, spirit of peppermint, and potassium carbonate in a simple syrup for many gastrointestinal issues. Glyconda was a preparation that combined these ingredients in glycerin instead of simple syrup; it was often used as a vehicle for other medicines.

Glycoside: Any of a group of organic compounds, occurring abundantly in plants, that yield a sugar and one or more nonsugar substances.

Grain: A unit of apothecary weight equal to one-sixtieth of a dram.

Hemoptysis: The expectoration of blood or of blood-streaked sputum from the larynx, trachea, bronchi, or lungs.

Hepar Sulphur: Liver of sulphur; a substance of a liver-brown color, sometimes used in medicine. It is formed by fusing sulphur with carbonates of the alkalis (esp. potassium), and consists essentially of alkaline sulphides. Called also *hepar sulphuris.*

Homeopathy: A medical system that operates on the principle that "like cures like." Homeopaths administer minute doses of remedies that cause the very symptoms that the patient is most troubled by.

Hyperemia: The presence of an increased amount of blood in a body part or organ.

Hyperesthesia: Abnormal acuteness of sensitivity to touch, pain, or other sensory stimuli.

Ichorous: Resembling watery pus

Icteric hue: Yellowish

Intercostal: Situated between the ribs.

Inotropic: Increasing the heart's beating strength - how hard it squeezes

In vitro: In an artificial environment, such as a test tube.

Laboratory Biosafety levels, BSL:
Biosafety Level 1 is suitable for work involving well-characterized agents not known to consistently cause disease in healthy adult humans, and of minimal potential hazard to laboratory personnel and the environment.;
Biosafety Level 2 is similar to Biosafety Level 1 and is suitable for work involving agents of moderate potential hazard to personnel and the environment. It differs from BSL-1 in that (1) laboratory personnel have specific training in handling pathogenic agents and are directed by competent scientists;
Biosafety Level 3 is applicable to clinical, diagnostic, teaching, research, or production facilities in which work is done with indigenous or exotic agents which may cause serious or potentially lethal disease as a result of exposure by the inhalation route. Laboratory personnel have specific training in handling pathogenic and potentially lethal agents, and are supervised by competent scientists who are experienced in working with these agents;
Biosafety Level 4 is required for work with dangerous and exotic agents that pose a high individual risk of aerosol-transmitted laboratory infections and life-threatening disease. Agents with a close or identical antigenic relationship to Biosafety Level 4 agents are handled at this level until sufficient data are obtained either to confirm continued work at this level, or to work with them at a lower level. Members of the laboratory staff have specific and thorough training in handling extremely hazardous infectious agents and they understand the primary and secondary containment functions of the standard and special practices, the containment equipment, and the laboratory design characteristics. They are supervised by competent scientists who are trained and experienced in working with these agents. Access to the laboratory is strictly controlled by the laboratory director. For further details: http://www.cdc.gov/od/ohs/biosfty/bmbl4/bmbl4s3.htm

Lactucarium: Concrete milk juice of *Lactuca virosa* (bitter lettuce). It is obtained by cutting the stems at the time of flowering, soaking up the milky juice that flows out with a sponge or cotton and then squeezing it out into a vessel containing a little water. This mixture is left in a dry place until it solidifies into a solid mass. Multiple sequential cuts are made a short distance below the first several times daily until all of the plant juice has been collected.

Leucocytes: "White cells" - a broad term referring to the white cell population of the blood, including B cells, T cells, monocytes, macrophages, basophils, eosinophils, neutrophils, and NK cells. While in the bloodstream, many of these cells are relatively undifferentiated (immature) and only activated at the site of an infection, once exposed to an antigen.

Low dose (or drop dose) herb: An herb that can be used safely in very low doses but may be toxic at higher doses.

Mastitis: Inflammation of the breast.

Materia medica: The scientific study of medicinal drugs and their sources, preparation, and use.

Meningitis: Inflammation of the meninges of the brain and the spinal cord, most often caused by a bacterial or viral infection and characterized by fever, vomiting, intense headache, and stiff neck.

Minim: A unit of fluid measure, as: In the United States, a minim is one-sixtieth of a fluid dram (0.0616 milliliters) and in Great Britain, a minim is one-twentieth of a scruple (0.0592 milliliters).

Myalgia: Muscular pain or tenderness, especially when diffuse and nonspecific.

Nephritis: Any of various acute or chronic inflammations of the kidneys, such as Bright's disease.

Nervine: An agent that calms nervousness, tension or excitement.

Neuralgia: A sharp, shooting pain along a nerve pathway.

Orchitis: Inflammation of the testicles.

Osteopath: A system of medicine based on the theory that disturbances in the musculoskeletal system affect other bodily parts, causing many disorders that can be corrected by various manipulative techniques in conjunction with conventional medical, surgical, pharmacological, and other therapeutic procedures.

Otitis media: A middle ear infection. Fluid can be present with or without infection, and may cause temporary hearing loss that can evolve into permanent loss.

Papillae: Small bumps (papillae) cover the upper surface of the tongue. Between the papillae are the taste buds, which provide the sense of taste.

Paroxysmal: Recurring "sudden attacks" of symptoms, whooping cough is a paroxysmal cough.

Pertussin: Pertussin is a brand of cough syrup that contains dextromorphan. It is used to relieve coughs due to colds or influenza. It should not be used for chronic cough that occurs with smoking, asthma, or emphysema or when there is an unusually large amount of mucus or phlegm (also flem) with the cough.

Pharynx: The hollow tube about five inches long that starts behind the nose and ends at the top of the trachea (windpipe) and esophagus (the tube that goes to the stomach). The pharyngeal tissue lines the pharynx.

Physic: A purging medicine that stimulates evacuation of the bowels

Phytotherapist: A health care practitioner who uses plant medicines to treat patients.

Pleurisy: Inflammation of the membranes surrounding the lungs.

Pleuritis: An inflammation of the pleura, the thin covering that protects and cushions the lungs. When the pleura become inflamed, more than a normal amount of fluid can be produced, causing a pleural effusion.

Potassium citrate: An aqueous liquid containing in solution about nine percent anhydrous potassium citrate together with small amounts of citric and carbonic acids. The solution is a refrigerant acting mildly on the skin, bowels, and kidneys. It is very useful in allaying gastric irritability. Its sedative and diaphoretic properties may be augmented by the addition of aconite or of digitalis. Its diuretic influence is rendered more certain by combining it with sweet spirit of niter. In diarrhea or irritable bowels, some opium or morphine may be added to it. It forms "a very grateful draught" for fever patients and may be sweetened with sugar if needed. The dose is one tablespoonful, diluted with about an equal measure of water and repeated five or six or more times in the course of a day. A similar preparation may be given as an effervescent drink by forming one solution of lemon juice and water (each one-half fluid ounce) and another by dissolving bicarbonate of potassium, one and one-half drams in four ounces of water. The two solutions are mixed and taken during the effervescence.

Precordial: Pertaining to the region over the heart and stomach.

Prophylactic: A preventative

Ptosis: Drooping of the eyelids.

Puerperal: Period following childbirth

Puerperal eclampsia: Convulsions and coma associated with hypertension, oedema, or proteinuria occurring in a woman following delivery.

Purulent meningitis: Meningitis is an infection that causes inflammation of the membranes covering the brain and spinal cord. Non-bacterial meningitis is often referred to as "aseptic meningitis." Bacterial meningitis may be referred to as "purulent meningitis."

Purulent: Having or making pus

Rales: Clicking, bubbling or rattling sounds that occur when air moves through fluid-filled airways

Regular: A physician who practices allopathic or mainstream medicine.

Sclera: The white, protective, outer layer of the eyeball.

Seidlitz powder: A gentle laxative. Put two drams of tartrate potassium and sodium together with 40 grains of sodium bicarbonate in a blue paper and 35 grains of tartaric acid in a white paper. Dissolve the powders in two half tumblers of water, mix and drink immediately while effervescing. A simpler but very satisfactory alternative is to mix two parts of sodium bitartrate with one part sodium bicarbonate. This powder keeps well and effervesces briskly when mixed with water. The powder is named after the Seidlitz Saline Springs in Bohemia although the constituents do not represent those of those springs. This is a very popular laxative, especially where there is a slight rise of temperature and particularly in warm weather. The mixture should be used with care in very young children and the elderly or debilitated. Under no circumstances should one solution be swallowed after the other because the liberation of carbon dioxide in the stomach gives rise to serious distension if not rupture of the stomach.

Septicemia: Disease caused by the spread of bacteria and their toxins in the bloodstream. Also called blood poisoning.

Serous tissue: A thin membrane lining the closed cavities of the body; has two layers with a space between that is filled with serous fluid, normal lymph of a serous cavity

Sialagogue: Promotes the flow of saliva.

Sinapism: Mustard plaster, applied to the skin as a counter-irritant.

Sodium hyposulphite: It was used to deodorize fermentative and putrefactive changes within or without the body. It was used for its deodorizing property in pulmonary gangrene and fetid bronchitis, and was said to often cure the latter. A syrup was often prepared for internal use using one dram of hyposulphite and two ounces seven drams of sugar and one and one-half ounces of water, dissolved with gentle heat. Dose: One to four tablespoons. A bath was prepared by adding one to four ounces of the salt to the bathwater.

Sordes: Foul matter; excretion; dregs; filthy, useless, or rejected matter of any kind. Specifically, the foul matter that collects on the teeth and tongue in low fevers and other conditions attended with great vital depression.

Sthenic fever: Strong or active fever, especially of morbid states attended with excessive action of the heart and blood vessels, and characterized by strength and activity of the muscular and nervous system.

Sthenic: Relating to or marked by sthenia; strong, vigorous, or active.

Sudiferous glands: Sweat producing structures that are embedded in the skin.

Syrup of coccilana: Cocillana bark comes from a Brazilian tree, *Syocarpus rusbyi*. Its action closely resembles that of ipecac. In doses of ten to 20 drops of a fluid extract, it was reported to be effective in acute and chronic bronchial ailments. It was not widely used by the Eclectics.

Syrup of Squill: Also known as hive or cough syrup. It combines *Urginea maritima* (squill), *Polygala senega* (Senega snakeroot), antimony, and potassium tartrate in a syrup. It was not used by the Eclectics.

Syrupus Aurantii (Orange syrup): A very slight sedative effect is produced by this syrup in delicate individuals whose nervous system is easily excited. Its chief use, however, is in flavoring other medicines.

Tepid or warm sponge bath: This is exceedingly useful in many febrile conditions. The skin is relaxed and the radiation of heat is not prevented as by immersion. Sponging the head constantly with warm water, drawing the sponge back and forth and, at the same time, fanning the person is far more effective and safe than is local application of cold water or ice, which probably does little more than chill the surface. (tepid means 29.4 to 33.3 degrees Celsius or 85 to 92 degrees Fahrenheit).

Tincture: A plant extracted in water and alcohol.

Tobacco heart: A rapid, irregular heart rate resulting from excessive use of tobacco.

Transcutaneous: Transdermal,: through the unbroken skin.

Trigeminal neuralgia: Sharp shooting lancinating pain found in the forehead, face or jaw region.

Triturition: Trituration is the grinding of powders in a mortar with a pestle.

Typhoid character: Typhoid fever is an acute illness with fever caused by infection by the *Salmonella typhii* bacteria from contaminated water and food. The disease has an insidious onset characterized by fever, headache, constipation, malaise, chills, and myalgia (muscle pain). Diarrhea is uncommon, and vomiting is not usually severe. Confusion, delirium, intestinal perforation, and death may occur in severe cases. A disease of a typhoid character would cause similar symptoms.

Vagal: Of or relating to a nerve that helps control function of the esophagus, voice box (larynx), stomach, intestines, lungs and heart.

Vesicular: A small sac or cyst, especially one containing fluid.

Widal: A test of blood serum that uses an agglutination reaction to diagnose typhoid fever.

Zinc Chloride: Large doses of zinc chloride act as an irritant poison, producing a burning sensation in the stomach, nausea, vomiting, anxiety, short breathing, small quick pulse, cold sweats, fainting, and convulsions. In small doses it has been given in scrofula, chorea, epilepsy and other nervous diseases. It is now seldom employed as an internal medicine. It is used topically as an escharotic, a caustic substance that destroys tissue and causes sloughing.

Appendix B

Summary of the responses of 222 physicians to the Lloyd Brothers' survey tabulating how many physicians listed an herb as most useful (1st Place) and how many listed it as one of the six most useful (Top Six).

Remedy	1st Place	Top Six	Remedy	1st Place	Top Six
Gelsemium	68	193	Drosera	1	3
Aconite	52	170	Gelsemium/ Echinacea	1	
Eupatorium	30	92	Gelsemium/ Actea	1	
Bryonia	19	162	Phenacetin	1	1
Veratrum	10	87	Iris	1	1
Actea racemosa	9	114	Eupatorium/ Gel/cactus	1	
Lobelia	8	79	Cactus	0	64
Belladonna	5	48	Ipecac	0	57
Echinacea	5	29	Sanguinaria	0	34
Gelsemium/ Aconite	3		Rhus	0	25
Asclepias	3	72	Euphrasia	0	10
Aconite/ Eupatorium	2		Nux vomica	0	9

Remedy	1st Place	Top Six	Remedy	1st Place	Top Six
Bicarbonate	1	1	Phytolacca	0	8
Aconite/ Echinacea	1		Baptisia	0	6
Sodium salicylate	0	6	Sticta	0	3
Digitalis	0	5	Calcium	1	
Quinine	0	5	Cactus sulfite	0	2
Stillingia	0	5	Cinnamon	0	2
Aspirin	0	4	Codeine	0	2
Collinsonia	0	4	Hydrastis	0	2
Jaborandi	0	4	Hyocyamus	0	2
Sodium sulfate	0	4	Mur Amm	0	2
Sodium sulfite	0	4	Am carb	0	1
Podophyllin	0	4	Apis	0	1
Calomel	0	3	Apocynum	0	1
Castor oil	0	3	Arnica	0	1
Nitre spirits	0	3	Avena	0	1
Pulsatilla	0	3	Berberine	0	1
Br pot	0	1	Iodine	0	1
Calcium iodide	0	1	Kali Mur	0	1

Remedy	1st Place	Top Six	Remedy	1st Place	Top Six
Caffeine	0	1	Lemonade	0	1
Cannabis	0	1	Lime I	0	1
Cinchinoid	0	1	Mercuric	0	1
Cinnamon/ sassafras	0	1	Morphine	0	1
Corydalis	0	1	Sodium citrate	0	1
Dioscorea	0	1	Passiflora	0	1
Emetic tincture	0	1	Peppermint essence	0	1
Erigeron	0	1	Phenacetin	0	1
Hamamelis	0	1	Pilocarpine	0	1
Hepar sulfate	0	1	Potassium chloride	0	1
Heroin	0	1	Scutellaria	0	1
Hot water	0	1	Senega	0	1
Serpentaria	0	1	Squill's syrup	0	1
Spongia	0	1	Sodium sulfide	0	1
Spirits of ammonia	0	1	Trifolium	0	1

Several responders identified two or more herbs as most important. These herbs are included in the total for each of those herbs but are not added to the number of the single most important choice.

APPENDIX C
Tincture Sources

Many companies prepare and sell herbal tinctures to the public, and their product lines will contain some of the plants discussed in this book. The following are only a few of those companies. Most prepare tinctures from fresh plants, and are run by trained herbalists.

Herbalist & Alchemist
51 S. Wandling Ave.
Washington, NJ 07882
http://www.herbalist-alchemist.com/

Herb Pharm
P.O. Box 116
Williams, Oregon 97544
http://www.herb-pharm.com/

Herbs Etc.
1340 Rufina Circle
Santa Fe, NM 87507
http://www.herbsetc.com/

Vitality Works
8409 Washington St NE
Albuquerque, NM. 87113
http://www.vitalityworks.com/vitality/about.htm

Low Dose Tinctures

Low dose herbs are only available to trained or licensed professionals. Further, due to low demand and insurance issues, many low dose herbs used by the Eclectics simply are not available at all in commerce. The following company sells low dose herbal tinctures to trained or licensed professionals only:

Heron Botanicals
26013 United Rd. NE #210
Poulsbo, WA 98370
www.heronbotanicals.com

On occasion, some of the other tincture companies listed above may sell some low dose tinctures to trained professionals although they do not advertise that they do.

Locating a Professional Practitioner

In 1918, the Eclectic physicians were trained in medicine and in the use of plants to treat serous illness. They had much experience using plants in difficult diseases such as pneumonia. Many Eclectics practicing in 1918 also treated patients during the 1889-1890 pandemic. When the 1918 pandemic hit, they already had hands-on experience in treating pandemic influenza. Younger Eclectic physicians had the advantage of being trained by physicians who had used plant remedies with success in pandemic influenza.

Today, few physicians are taught how to use plants at all, let alone how to use them in pandemic influenza. The few who use botanicals typically only know the most commonly used medicinal plants. As a general rule, only licensed naturopathic physicians and professional herbalists will have experience in using many of the plants described by the Eclectics for influenza. None will have experience in treating pandemic influenza but many will have treated seasonal influenza with herbs. Anyone who may want access to Eclectic treatments during a pandemic should consider establishing a relationship with a qualified professional now. The American Association of Naturopathic Physicians (AANP) and the American Herbalists Guild (AHG) maintain websites where professional practitioners can be located.

The American Association of Naturopathic Physicians was founded in 1985. It is the national professional society representing naturopathic physicians "NDs" who are licensed, or eligible for licensing, as primary care providers. Licensed naturopathic physicians attend a four-year graduate level naturopathic medical school. They are educated in all of the same basic sciences as an M.D. but, in addition to the standard medical curriculum, also complete four years of training in clinical nutrition, acupuncture, homeopathic medicine, botanical medicine, psychology, and counseling. A naturopathic physician must pass a professional board exam in order to be licensed as a primary care general practice physician.

The American Association of Naturopathic Physicians
4435 Wisconsin Avenue, NW Suite 403, Washington, DC 20016
Email: member.services@Naturopathic.org
Website: Http://www.naturopathic.org

The American Herbalists Guild was founded in 1989, and is the only peer-reviewed organization in the United States for professional herbalists specializing in the medicinal use of plants. Their website lists all practitioners who meet their criteria for professional membership in the AHG.

The American Herbalists Guild
141 Nob Hill Road, Cheshire, CT 06410
Email: ahgoffice@earthlink.net
Website: http://www.americanherbalistsguild.com

References

[1] http://www.cdc.gov/flu/avian/gen-info/transmission.htm July 2006

[2] La grippe—its history, causes and types. *Eclectic Medical Journal* 1915; 75(2):98-101.

[3] Barry JM. *The Great Influenza* NY NY Penguin Books 2005.

[4] Barry JM. *The Great Influenza* NY NY Penguin Books 2005.

[5] Barry JM. *The Great Influenza* NY NY Penguin Books 2005.

[6] Rudd RT. Influenza and its treatment. *Eclectic Medical Journal* 1920; 80(8):377-379.

[7] Small WDD, Blanchard WO. The treatment of influenza. *Eclectic Medical Journal* 1919; 79(8):444-446.

[8] Kitsmiller CR. Influenza. *Eclectic Medical Journal* 1918; 78(4):179-181.

[9] Holtzmuller CW. Pneumonia following influenza. *Eclectic Medical Journal* 1920; 80(1):15-16.

[10] Holtzmuller CW. Pneumonia following influenza. *Eclectic Medical Journal* 1920; 80(1):15-16.

[11] http://www.who.int/mediacentre/factsheets/avian_influenza/en/#case April 2006

[12] http://www.who.int/mediacentre/factsheets/avian_influenza/en/#case April 2006

[13] http://www.cdc.gov/nip/vacsafe/concerns/gbs/default.htm July 2006

[14] http://www.mainehealthforum.org/ShowARticle.asp?aid=6258&rid=365 July 2006

[15] http://www.fda.gov/cder/foi/nda/99/21087_Tamiflu_pharmr_P2.pdf July 2006

[16] http://www.fda.gov/cder/foi/nda/99/21087_Tamiflu_pharmr_P1.pdf July 2006

[17] http://www.fda.gov/cder/foi/nda/99/021036-medreview1.pdf July 2006

[18] http://bioterrorism.slu.edu/AvianJune05/OurBestShot.pdf July 2006

[19] http://www.whitehouse.gov/homeland/nspi_implementation.pdf July 2006

[20] http://www.fda.gov/cdrh/ppe/fluoutbreaks.html#12 July 2006

[21] http://www.kansascity.com/mld/kansascity/business/14357980.htm July 2006

[22] http://www.kansascity.com/mld/kansascity/business/14357980.htm July 2006

[23] Miller HI. Flummoxing the Flu, We need many parallel strategies. http://www.nationalreview.com/comment/miller200511020858.asp July

2006

[24] http://www.democrats.reform.house.gov/Documents/20041018110107-30762.pdf July 2006

[25] http://www.coxwashington.com/reporters/content/reporters/stories/BC_VACCINE_LIABILITY11_COX.html July 2006.

[26] Barry J. The Great Influenza. New York, NY Penguin Books 2004.

[27] Griggs B. Green Pharmacy, the history and evolution of Western herbal medicine. Rochester VT Healing Arts Press 1997.

[28] Griggs B. "Green Pharmacy" Rochester VT Healing Arts Press 1997.

[29] Collins AJ. What is Eclecticism? Http://www.planetherbs.com/articles/eclectics.html April 2006.

[30] Collins AJ. What is Eclecticism? Http://www.planetherbs.com/articles/eclectics.html April 2006.

[31] Moore M. Introduction to the National Eclectic Medical Association Quarterly. Http://www.swsbm.com/quarterlies/quarterly.htm May 2006.

[32] Anon. Increase in women doctors changing the face of medicine. http://www.nejmjobs.org/rpt/increase-in-women-drs.aspx June 2006.

[33] Steinreich D. 100 years of medical robbery. Townsend Letter for Doctors & Patients 2004; Oct. Available at http://findarticles.com June 2006

[34] Hiatt MD. Around the continent in 180 days: The controversial journey of Abraham Flexner. The Pharos Winter 1999

[35] Hiatt MD. Around the continent in 180 days: The controversial journey of Abraham Flexner. The Pharos Winter 1999

[36] Flexner Report. http://www.carnegiefoundation.org/publications June 2006.

[37] Hiatt MD. Around the continent in 180 days: The controversial journey of Abraham Flexner. The Pharos Winter 1999.

[38] Collins AJ. What is Eclecticism? Http://www.planetherbs.com/articles/eclectics.html April 2006.

[39] Feikin Dr, Schuchat A, Kolczak M, et al. Mortality from invasive pneumococcal pneumonia in the era of antibiotic resistance, 1995-1997. Am J Publ Health 2000; 90(2):223-229.

[40] Small WDD, Blanchard WO. The treatment of influenza. Eclectic Medical Journal 1919; 79(8):444-446.

[41] Small WDD, Blanchard WO. The treatment of influenza. Eclectic Medical Journal 1919; 79(8):444-446.

[42] http://www.spartacus.schoolnet.co.uk/FWWinfluenzia.htm July 2006.

[43] Scudder JM. *Specific Medication and Specific Medicines.* (10th Ed.) Cincinnati, OH Wilstach, Baldwind & Co. 1881.

[44] McGuffin M, Hobbs C, Upton R, Goldberg A. *American Herbal Products Association's Botanical Safety Handbook.* Boca Raton FL CRC Press 1997.

[45] Chan MCW, Cheung CY, Chui WH, et al. Proinflammatory cytokine responses induced by influenza A (H5N1) viruses in primary human

alveolar and bronchial epithelial cells. *Resp Res* 2005; 6(1):135-147

[46] Sharma M, Arnason JT, Burt A, Hudson JR. Echinacea extracts modulate the pattern of chemokine and cytokine secretion in rhinovirus-infected and uninfected epithelial cells. *Phytother Res* 2006; 20(2):147-152.

[47] Scudder JM. *Specific Medication and Specific Medicines.* (10th Ed.) Cincinnati, OH Wilstach, Baldwind & Co. 1881.

[48] Mitchell WA Jr. *Plant Medicine in Practice.* St. Louis MO Churchill Livingstone 2003

[49] Felter HW. *The Eclectic Materia Medica, Pharmacology and Therapeutics* Sandy OR Eclectic Medical Publications 1983.

[50] Felter HW, Lloyd JU. King's American Dispensatory Sandy OR Eclectic Medical Publications 1993.

[51] Hoffmann D. *Medical Herbalism.* Rochester VT Healing Arts Press 2003.

[52] Moerman DE. *Native American Ethnobotany.* Portland, OR Timber Press 1998.

[53] Weiss RF. *Weiss's Herbal Medicine Classic Edition* NY NY Thieme 2001

[54] Blue R. (Surgeon General) "Spanish influenza." *Eclectic Medical Journal* 1918; 78(11):561-563.

[55] Anon. Prophylaxis and treatment of influenza and influenzal pneumonia. *Eclectic Medical Journal* 1919; 79(12):670.

[56] Weiss RF. *Weiss's Herbal Medicine Classic Edition* NY NY Thieme 2001.

[57] Mitchell WA Jr. *Plant Medicine in Practice.* St. Louis MO Churchill Livingstone 2003

[58] McGuffin M, Hobbs C, Upton R, Goldberg R. *American Herbal Products Association's Botanical Safety Handbook* Boca Raton FL CRC Press 1997.

[59] Felter HW. Epidemic influenza. *Eclectic Medical Journal* 1899; 59(1):42-45.

[60] Eclectic Medication in la grippe. *Eclectic Medical Journal* 1915; 75(2):98-103.

[61] Influenza again. *Eclectic Medical Journal* 191; 79(10):557.

[62] Some influenza suggestions. *Eclectic Medical Journal* 1918; 78(11):604.

[63] Mitchell WA Jr. *Plant Medicine in Practice.* St. Louis MO Churchill Livingstone 2003

[64] Hoffmann D. *Medical Herbalism.* Rochester VT Healing Arts Press 2003.

[65] Mills S, Bone K. *Principles and Practice of Phytotherapy.* NY, NY Srchill Livingstone 2000.

[66] Blumenthal M, Goldberg A, Brinckmann J. *Herbal Medicine Expanded Commission E Monographs.* Newton MA Integrative Medicine Communications 2000.

[67] Felter HW, Lloyd JU. King's American Dispensatory Sandy OR Eclectic Medical Publications 1993.

[68] Felter HW. *The Eclectic Materia Medica, Pharmacology and Therapeutics* Sandy OR Eclectic Medical Publications 1983.

[69] The pharynx in influenza. *Eclectic Medical Journal* 1906; 66(11):544.

[70] Influenza again. *Eclectic Medical Journal* 1919; 79(10):530-531.

[71] Mundy WN. Valuable remedies for influenza, grippe, and "common colds." http://www.herbaltherapeutics.net/herbal_therapeutics_library.htm June 2006.

[72] Hoffmann D. *Medical Herbalism.* Rochester VT Healing Arts Press 2003.

[73] Moore M. *Medicinal Plants of the Mountain West.* (revised and expanded edition). *Santa Fe NM* Museum of New Mexico Press 2003.

[74] Mills S, Bone K. *Principles and Practice of Phytotherapy.* NY, NY Churchill Livingstone 2000.

[75] Mitchell WA Jr. *Plant Medicine in Practice.* St. Louis MO Churchill Livingstone 2003.

[76] Moore M. *Medicinal Plants of the Mountain West.* (revised and expanded edition). *Santa Fe NM* Museum of New Mexico Press 2003.

[77] Felter HW. Epidemic influenza. *Eclectic Medical Journal* 1899; 59(1):142-145.

[78] Bowles T, Harrison O. Remedies I employ in treating influenza. *Eclectic Medical Journal* 1920: 80(12):595-598.

[79] Influenza in children. *Eclectic Medical Journal* 1922; 82(8):407-408.

[80] Veratrum viride monograph by WE Daniels, MD, Madison SD *Ellingwood Therapeutist.*

[81] Mitchell WA Jr. *Plant Medicine in Practice.* St. Louis MO Churchill Livingstone 2003

[82] Personal communication with Michael Moore, 1998.

[83] Goetz P. [Phytotherapie of headaches] [in French] *Phytother* 2005; 3(4):176-177.

[84] Weiss RF. *Weiss's Herbal Medicine Classic Edition* NY NY Thieme 2001.

[85] Lloyd JU. Gelsemium. http://www.swsbm.com/ManualsOther/Gelsemium-Lloyd.PDF April 2006.

[86] Felter HW. Epidemic influenza. *Eclectic Medical Journal* 1899; 59(1):42-45.

[87] Eclectic medication in la grippe. *Eclectic Medical Journal* 1915; 75(2):102-103.

[88] Influenza again. *Eclectic Medical Journal* 1919; 79(10):557

[89] Bowles T, Harrison O. Remedies I employ in treating influenza. *Eclectic Medical Journal* 1920: 80(12):595-598.

[90] Moerman DE. *Native American Ethnobotany.* Portland, OR Timber Press 1998.

[91] Weiss RF. *Weiss's Herbal Medicine Classic Edition* NY NY Thieme 2001.

[92] Personal communication with Michael Moore, 1998.

[93] Mitchell WA Jr. *Plant Medicine in Practice.* St. Louis MO Churchill Livingstone 2003

[94] Bello-Ramirez AM, Nava-Ocampo AA. A QSAR analysis of Aconitum alkaloids. *Fund Clin Pharmacol* 2004; 18(6):699-704.

[95] Kim IT, Park SK, Shin JP, et al. The efficacy of methylprednisolone in

aconite-induced myelo-optic neuropathy in the rabbit. *Neuro-Ophthamol* 2000; 24(1):301-310.

[96] Braca A, Fico G, Morelli I, et al. Antioxidant and free radical scavenging activity of flavonol glycosides from different Aconitum species. *J Ethnopharmacol* 2003; 86(1):63-67.

[97] Elliott SP. A case of fatal poisoning with aconite plant: Quantitative analysis in biological fluid. *Sci & Justice* 2002; 42(2):111-115.

[98] Dobbelstein H. [Attempted murder using aconitum. Background of a toxicological emergency.] [in German] *MMW Fortschr Med* 2000; 142(42):46-47.

[99] Tyrrell GG. The epidemic influenza. *Eclectic Medical Journal* 1873; 33(12):567-568.

[100] The grippe. *Eclectic Medical Journal* 1894; 44-45.

[101] Eclectic medication in la grippe. *Eclectic Medical Journal* 1915; 75(2):102-103.

[102] Some influenza suggestions. *Eclectic Medical Journal* 1918; 78(11):606.

[103] Rudd RT. Influenza and its treatment. *Eclectic Medical Journal* 1920; 80(8):377-379.

[104] *The Gleaner* 1926:27.

[105] Mundy WN. Valuable remedies for influenza, grippe, and "common colds." http://www.herbaltherapeutics.net/herbal_therapeutics_library.htm June 2006.

[106] Spanish Influenza. *Ellingwood's Therapeutist*

[107] Lloyd Brother survey http://www.herbaltherapeutics.net/herbal_therapeutics_library.htm June 2006

[108] Krieger HA. Influenza. *Ellingwood's Therapeutist.*

[109] Lloyd Brother survey http://www.herbaltherapeutics.net/herbal_therapeutics_library.htm June 2006.

[110] Lloyd Brother survey http://www.herbaltherapeutics.net/herbal_therapeutics_library.htm June 2006.

[111] Zagler B, Zelger A, Salvatore C, et al. Dietary poisoning with Veratrum album – a report of two cases. *Wiener Klinische Wochenschrift* 2005; 117(3):106-108.

[112] Prince LA, Stork CM. Prolonged cardiotoxicity from poison lily (Veratrum viride). *Vet & Human Toxicol* 2000; 42(5):282-285.

[113] Quatrehomme G, Bertrand F, Chauvet C, Ollier A. Intoxication form Veratrum album. *Human & Exp Toxicol* 1993; 12(2):111-115.

[114] Ventura HO, Mehra MR, Messerli FH. Desperate diseases, desperate measures: Tackling malignant hypertension in the 1950s. *Am Heart J* 2001; 142(2):197-203.

[115] Practial suggestions in the treatment of pneumonia. *Ellingwoods Therapeutist.*

[116] Daniels WE. Veratrum viride. *Ellingwood Therapeutist.*

[117] Daniels WE. Veratrum viride. *Ellingwood Therapeutist.*

[118] Bowles T, Harrison O. Remedies I employ in treating influenza. *Eclectic Medical Journal* 1920: 80(12):595-598.

[119] Park CS, Lim H, Han KJ, et al. Inhibition of nitric oxide generation by 23, 24-dihydrocucurbitacin D in mouse peritoneal macrophages. *J Pharmacol & Exp Ther* 2004; 309(2):705-710.

[120] La grippe in Australia. *Eclectic Medical Journal* 1892; 52(4):163-166.

[121] Felter HW. Epidemic influenza. *Eclectic Medical Journal* 1899; 59(1):42-45.

[122] Some remedies in influenza. *Ellingwoods Therapeutist* :524.

[123] The pharynx in influenza. *Eclectic Medical Journal* 1906; 66(11):544.

[124] Eclectic medication in la grippe. *Eclectic Medical Journal* 1915; 75(2):102-103.

[125] *Eclectic Medical Journal* 1915; 75(2):98-103.

[126] Bowles T, Harrison O. Remedies I employ in treating influenza. *Eclectic Medical Journal* 1920: 80(12):595-598.

[127] Practical suggestions in the treatment of pneumonia. *Ellingwoods Therapeutist*.

[128] Bowles T, Harrison O. Remedies I employ in treating influenza. *Eclectic Medical Journal* 1920: 80(12):595-598

[129] Griggs B. *"Green Pharmacy"* Rochester VT Healing Arts Press 1997.

[130] Subarnas A, Oshima Y, Sidik, Ohizumi Y. An antidepressant principle of Lobelia inflata L. (Campanulaceae). *J Pharmaceut Sci* 1992; 81(7):620-621.

[131] Subarnas A, Tadano T, Nakahata N, et al. A possible mechanism of antidepressant activity of beta-amyrin palmitate isolated from Lobelia inflata leaves in the forced swimming test. *Life Sci* 1993; 52(3):289-296.

[132] Subarnas A, Tadano T, Oshima Y, et al. Pharmacological properties of beta-amyrin palmitate, a novel centrally acting compound, isolated from Lobelia inflata leaves. *J Pharm Pharmacol* 1993; 45(6):545-550.

[133] Felpin F-X, Lebreton J. History, chemistry and biology of alkaloids from Lobelia inflata. *Tetrahedron* 2004; 60(45):10127-10153.

[134] Bowles T, Harrison O. Remedies I employ in treating influenza. *Eclectic Medical Journal* 1920: 80(12):595-598

[135] Caksen H. Odabas D. Akbayram S. Cesur Yasar. Arslan S. Uner A. Oner AF. Deadly nightshade (Atropa belladonna) intoxication: An analysis of 49 children. *Hum Exp Toxicol* 2003; 22(12):665-668.

[136] Sheroziya OP, Ermishkin VV, Lukoshkova EV, et al. Changes in swallowing-related tachycardia and respiratory arrhythmia induced by modulation of tonic parasympathetic influences. *Neurophysiol* 2003; 35(6):434-444.

[137] Bettermann H, cysarz D, Portsteffen A, Kummell HC. Bimodal dose-dependent effect on autonomic, cardiac control after oral administration of Atropa belladonna. *Auton Neurosci Basic & Clin* 2001; 90(1-2):132-137.

[138] Bousta d, Soulimani R, Jarmouni I, et al. Neurotropic, immunological and gastric effects of low doses of Atropa belladonna L., Gelsemium sempervirens L. and Poumon histamine in stressed mice. *J Ethnopharmacol*

2001; 74(3):205-215.

[139] Della Loggia R, Tubaro A, Redaelli C. [Evaluation of the activity on the mouse CNS of several plant extracts and a combination of them.] [in Italian]. *Riv Neurol* 1981; 51(5):297-310.

[140] Felter HW. *The Eclectic Materia Medica, Pharmacology and Therapeutics* Sandy OR Eclectic Medical Publications 1983.

[141] Practical suggestions in the treatment of pneumonia. *Ellingwoods Therapeutist.*

[142] Krieger HA Influenza. *Ellingood's Therapeutist*

[143] Scudder JM. *Specific Medication and Specific Medicines.* (10th Ed.) Cincinnati, OH Wilstach, Baldwind & Co. 1881.

[144] Duke JA. The Green Pharmacy Herbal Handbook. Rodale Emmaus, PA. 2000.

[145] Pizzorno JE Jr, Murray MT. *Textbook of Natural Medicine Third Edition.* St. Louis MO Churchill Livingstone 2006.

[146] Blumenthal M, Goldberg A & Brinckmann J. Herbal Medicine, Expanded Commission E Monographs. Integrative Medicine Communications Newton MA. 2000.

[147] Webster HT. Reflections on the treatment of influenza. *Eclectic Medical Journal* 1919; 79(4):188-190.

[148] Cox HT. Echinacea in influenza. *Eclectic Medical Journal* 1929; 89(8):529-531.

[149] Cox HT. A review of influenza. *Eclectic Medical Journal* 1931; 91(8):304-307.

[150] Anon. Committee for Veterinary Medicinal Products, Selenicereus grandiflorus, summary report. *The European Agency for the Evaluation of Medicinal Products, Veterinary Medicines Evaluation Unit* April 1999.

[151] Anon. Committee for Veterinary Medicinal Products, Selenicereus grandiflorus, summary report. *The European Agency for the Evaluation of Medicinal Products, Veterinary Medicines Evaluation Unit* April 1999.

[152] Hapke, H. J.; Strathmann, W. [Pharmacological effects of hordenine.] [In German] *DTW (Deutsche Tieraerztliche Wochenschrift)* 1995; 102 (6) : 228-232.

[153] Lin RC, Peyroux J, Seguin E, Koch M. Hypertensive effect of glycosidic derivatives of hordenine isolated from Selaginella doederleinii hieron and structural analogues in rats. *Phytother Res* 1991; 5(4):188-190.

[154] Lloyd JU. Cactus grandiflorus. http://www.swsbm.com/ManualsOther/Selenicereus-Lloyd.PDF July 2006.

[155] La grippe in Australia. *Eclectic Medical Journal* 1892; 52(4):163-166.

[156] After influenza. *Eclectic Medical Journal* 1919; 79(4):216-221

[157] Lloyd Brother survey http://www.herbaltherapeutics.net/herbal_therapeutics_library.htm June 2006.

[158] Lloyd Brother survey http://www.herbaltherapeutics.net/herbal_therapeutics_library.htm June 2006.

[159] Lloyd Brother survey http://www.herbaltherapeutics.net/herbal_

therapeutics_library.htm June 2006.

[160] Hoffmann D. *Medical Herbalism.* Rochester VT Healing Arts Press 2003.

[161] Axelsson P, Thorn SE, Wattwil M. Betamethasone does not prevent nausea and vomiting induced by ipecacuanha. *Acta Anaesthesiol Scand* 2004; 48(10):1283-1286.

[162] Cooper M, Sologuren A, Valiente R, Smith J. Effects of lerisetron, a new 5-HT3 receptor antagonist on ipecacuanha-induced emesis in healthy volunteers. *Arzneimittel Forsch* 2002; 52(9):689-694.

[163] Eclectic medication in la grippe. *Eclectic Medical Journal* 1915; 75(2):102-103.

[164] Lloyd Brother survey http://www.herbaltherapeutics.net/herbal_therapeutics_library.htm June 2006.

[165] Eun J-P, Koh GY. Suppression of angiogenesis by the plant alkaloid, sanginarine. *Biochem & Biophys Res Comm* 2004; 317(2):618-624.

[166] Adhami VM, Aziz MH, Reagan-Shaw SR, et al. Saguinarine causes cell cycle blockade and apoptosis of human prostate carcinoma cells via modulation of cylin kinase inhibitor-cyclin-cyclin-dependent kinase machinery. *Mol Cancer Ther* 2004; 3(8):933-940.

[167] Moerman DE *Native American Ethnobotany.* Portland, OR Timber Press *.

[168] Stevens FA. Status of poison ivy extracts. *JAMA* 1945; 127:912-921.

[169] Cardinali C, Francalanei S, Giomi B, et al. Systemic contact dermatitis from herbal and homeopathic preparations used for herpes virus treatment. *Acta Derm Venereol* 2004; 84(3):223-226.

[170] Cardinali C, Francalanei S, Giomi B, et al. Systemic contact dermatitis from herbal and homeopathic preparations used for herpes virus treatment. *Acta Derm Venereol* 2004; 84(3):223-226.

[171] Choi JY, Park CS, Choi J, et al. Cytotoxic effect of urushiol on human ovarian cancer cells. *J Microbiol Biotechnol* 2001; 11(3):399-405.

[172] Schneider I, Bucar F. Lipoxygenase inhibitors from natural plant sources. Part 1: Medicinal plants with inhibitory activity on arachidonate 5-lipoxygenase and 5-lipoxygenase/cyclooxygenase. *Phtytother Res* 2005; 19(2):91-102.

[173] Eclectic medication in la grippe. *Eclectic Medical Journal* 1915; 75(2):102-103.

[174] Rudd RT. Influenza and its treatment. *Eclectic Medical Journal* 1920; 80(8):377-379.

[175] Scudder JM. *Specific Medication and Specific Medicines.* (10th Ed.) Cincinnati, OH Wilstach, Baldwind & Co. 1881.

[176] Felter HW. Epidemic influenza. *Eclectic Medical Journal* 1899; 59(1):42-45.

[177] Felter HW. Epidemic influenza. *Eclectic Medical Journal* 1899; 59(1):42-45.

[178] Dawley MW. Influenza. *Eclectic Medical Journal* 1919; 79(10):530-531.

[179] Bowles T, Harrison O. Remedies I employ in treating influenza. *Eclectic Medical Journal* 1920: 80(12):595-598

[180] Moses FW. Some peculiar phases of the late epidemic of influenza. *Eclectic Medical Journal* 1929; 89(7):455-457.

[181] Naser B, Lund B, Henneicke-von Zepelin HH, et al. A randomized, double-blind, placebo-controlled, clinical dose-response trial of an extract of Baptisia, Echinacea and Thuja for the treatment of patients with common cold. *Phytomed* 2005; 12(10):715-722.

[182] Hauke W, Kohler G, Henneicke-von Zepelin HH, Freudenstein J. Esberitox N as a supportive therapy when providing standard antibiotic treatment in subjects with a severe bacterial infection (acute exacerbation of chronic bronchitis): A multicentric, prospective, double-blind, placebo-controlled study. *Chemother* 2002; 48(4-5):259-266.

[183] After Influenza. *Eclectic Medical Journal* 1919; 79(4):216-221.

[184] Spanish Influenza. *Ellingwoods Therapeutist.*

[185] Lloyd Brother survey http://www.herbaltherapeutics.net/herbal_therapeutics_library.htm June 2006..

[186] Lloyd Brother survey http://www.herbaltherapeutics.net/herbal_therapeutics_library.htm June 2006..

[187] Felter HW. Epidemic influenza. *Eclectic Medical Journal* 1899; 59(1):42-45.

[188] Bremser WE. Influenza *Ellingwood's Therapeutist*

[189] Weiss RF. *Weiss's Herbal Medicine Classic Edition* NY NY Thieme 2001..

[190] Mitchell WA Jr. *Plant Medicine in Practice.* St. Louis MO Churchill Livingstone 2003.

[191] La grippe in Australia. *Eclectic Medical Journal* 1892; 52(4):163-166.

[192] Webster HT. Reflections on the treatment of influenza. *Eclectic Medical Journal* 1919, 79(4):188-190.

[193] After influenza. *Eclectic Medical Journal* 1919; 79(4):216-221.

[194] Bowles T, Harrison O. Remedies I employ in treating influenza. *Eclectic Medical Journal* 1920: 80(12):595-598

[195] Bowles T, Harrison O. Remedies I employ in treating influenza. *Eclectic Medical Journal* 1920: 80(12):595-598

[196] Hasani A, Pavia D, Toms N, et al. Effect of aromatics on lung mucociliary clearance in patients with chronic airways obstruction. *J Alt Comp Med* 2003; 9(2):243-249.

[197] http://www.rxmed.com/b.main/b2.pharmaceutical/b2.1.monographs/CPS-%20Monographs/CPS-%20(General%20Monographs-%20A)/ANTIPHLOGISTINE%20RUB%20A.html April 2006.

[198] Petersen. FJ. Materia Medica and Clinical Therapeutics, 1905, http://www.henriettesherbal.com/eclectic/petersen/formula.html April 2006.

[199] Petersen. FJ. *Materia Medica and Clinical Therapeutics*, 1905, http://www.henriettesherbal.com/eclectic/petersen/formula.html April 2006.

[200] http://www.innvista.com/HEALTH/herbs/modeuse/poultice.htm April

2006

[201] Petersen. FJ. *Materia Medica and Clinical Therapeutics*, 1905, http://www.henriettesherbal.com/eclectic/petersen/formula.html April 2006.

[202] Http://en.wikipedia.org/wiki/aspirin March 2006

[203] Http://en.wikipedia.org/wiki/phenacetin March 2006

[204] The grippe. *Eclectic Medical Journal* 1894; 44-45

[205] Eclectic medication in la grippe. *Eclectic Medical Journal* 1915; 75(2):102-103

[206] Influenza again. *Eclectic Medical Journal* 1919; 79(10):557

[207] Petersen. FJ. *Materia Medica and Clinical Therapeutics*, 1905, http://www.henriettesherbal.com/eclectic/petersen/formula.html April 2006.

CPSIA information can be obtained
at www.ICGtesting.com
Printed in the USA
LVHW031143040520
654960LV00022B/2663